The 6-Week Plan to Harness Your Body's
Natural Rhythms to Lose Weight for Good!

THE Belly Melt DIET™

FROM THE THE EDITORS OF **Prevention**®

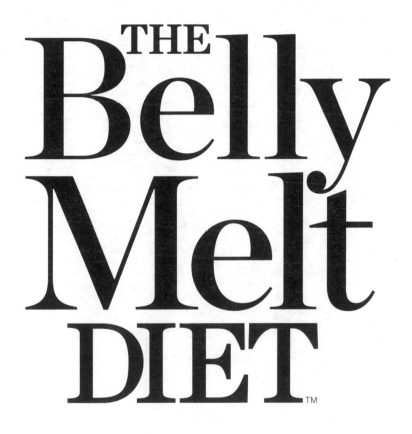

RODALE®

© 2012 by Rodale Inc.

Photographs © 2012 by Rodale Inc.

Success story portraits by Tom MacDonald/Rodale Images
Exercise photos by Mitch Mandel/Rodale Images

Library of Congress Cataloging-in-Publication Data
The editors of Prevention.
The belly melt diet: the 6-week plan to harness your body's natural rhythms to lose weight for good!/The editors of Prevention.
p.   cm.
Includes bibliographical references and index.
ISBN 978–1–60961–058–6   direct hardcover
1. Weight loss—Popular works.   2. Reducing exercise—Popular works.   3. Diet—Popular works.
4. Physical fitness—Popular works.   5. Self-care, Health—Popular works.
I. Prevention (Emmaus, Pa.)   II. Title.
RM222.2.D636   2012
613.7'12—dc23   2011037760

2   4   6   8   10   9   7   5   3   1   hardcover

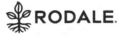

We inspire and enable people to improve their lives and the world around them.
For more of our products, visit prevention.com or call 800-848-4735.

Contents

Introduction

It's Time to Lose Weight for Good

If you're like most women, you've been fighting your body your entire adult life. You've beaten it up repeatedly with restrictive diets and brutal training regimes, perhaps losing weight, only to find that the pounds come right back after you tire of the impossible-to-keep-up-with diet and schedule. Then you blame yourself for a lack of willpower and your overwhelming desire to give in to cravings. It seems as if you're always fighting yourself.

This probably is no surprise to you: Americans—especially American women—spend millions of dollars on potions, pills, and programs that promise the body of their dreams, yet two out of three of us are overweight or obese. We slash calories, take up jogging, hire a personal trainer, and cut out every last gram of fat—yet it seems as though as soon as we lighten up a bit and try to return to a more "normal" way of eating and living, the pounds pack back on.

So what are you to do? Well, we're telling you to give up the fight.

Huh? That's right, by surrendering to your own understandable pattern of physical needs, and putting yourself in sync with your natural rhythms, you will finally flatten your belly and permanently win the war against weight gain.

It's time to establish a new cycle, one that doesn't involve weight falling off and piling on again. Food—and your relationship with food—is a huge part of it, of course. But what you put in your mouth depends more than you ever thought on the natural rhythms of life—circadian rhythms and how much sleep you get, the weather, your menstrual cycle, to say nothing of your stress and anxiety levels. Exercise matters, too, but that doesn't mean working out for the sake of working out. It means being aware that your body is ready to move more at certain times of the day—and that by working with your body's cycle instead of against it, you can burn more belly fat and build more metabolism-boosting lean muscle.

The Belly Melt Diet is the first weight-loss plan that takes into account how you feel and *why* you feel that way. Why do you want certain foods at certain times? Why do you eat more when you are tired? Why do you see better results when you work out at particular times of day? Answering these questions will allow you to make fitness and food choices that work in harmony with your body's needs. Our revolutionary weight loss plan will not only melt the belly fat right off you, but you will sleep better than ever, manage your stress like a champion, and never go hungry again in the quest for a slender figure.

The fight is over, and if you adopt this plan, you will be the lifetime winner of a toned and trim figure; you'll have more energy to do the things you love; and you'll possess a calm, focused mind that helps you get and stay in control of your physical and emotional self.

We'll Let You In on a Secret

What if we told you that we've discovered a secret? A secret that unlocks years of yo-yo dieting for a panel of women just like you, who are looking for a long-term solution not only to shed dangerous belly fat but to feel great, look younger, and reduce the risk of chronic diseases that make women old before their time.

The Belly Melt Diet is that secret. It's a plan based on who we really are as women. It's about embracing, not blaming, ourselves. Instead of counting calories, this revolutionary program teaches you to harness the power of your own internal cycles to lose weight, once and forever. This amazing new program seizes on the latest research of chronobiology—the study of biological rhythms—to show how the cycles in your life, from your daily eating patterns to your menstrual cycle to your sleep cycle, and even the seasons affect your appetite, cravings, moods, and, most important, weight loss.

The fact is, internal clocks govern nearly every aspect of our bodies, including the hormones that control appetite, metabolism, and fat storage. In *The Belly Melt Diet,* you'll learn to identify your own body rhythms and tweak the "master clock" in your brain to sync your cycles more to what experts say is ideal for reaching and maintaining a healthy weight. You're also going to learn why getting a good night's sleep is crucial to your ability to successfully lose weight—and keep it off.

Finally, we're going to give you a clear, doable step-by-step plan that will synchronize your rhythms to a more natural, healthful tempo that will maximize your fat-melting power. Follow the plan and we promise: You'll lose weight, sleep better, and have more energy to enjoy life to its fullest.

And if you don't believe us, you will believe the success stories of our Belly Melt test panel. This group of nine amazing women who followed the plan lost a total of 106 pounds and 57 inches (including 29 inches from just their waists) in 5 weeks! You'll read how they reset their body clocks to lose weight without feeling hungry and learned to get a good night's sleep, and they did it all without being stalked by cravings. You'll also read their tips and advice throughout the book so that we can help make their success *your* success.

Bottom line: You'll never be able to lose weight *and keep it off* until you learn to work with—not against—your natural rhythms. So let's get started.

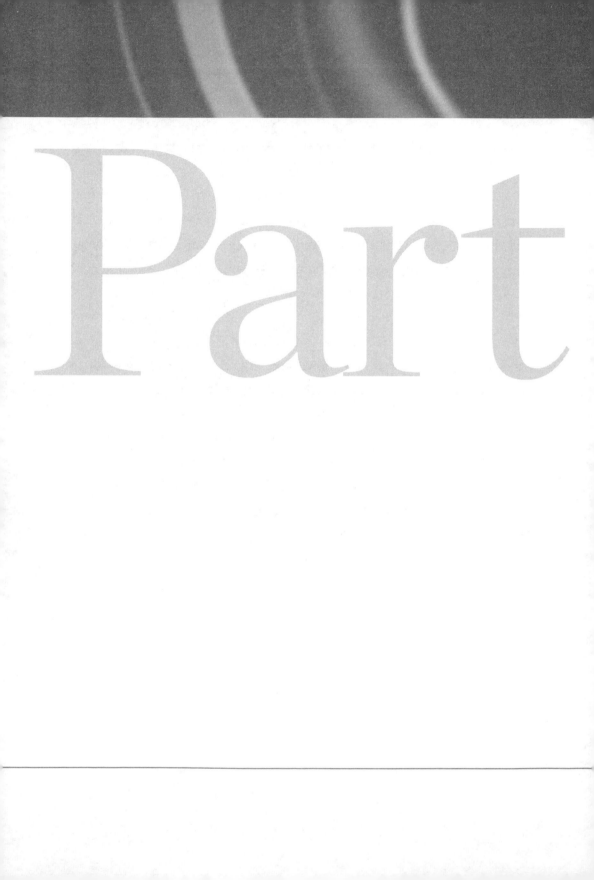

Part

I

The Body Clock Reset

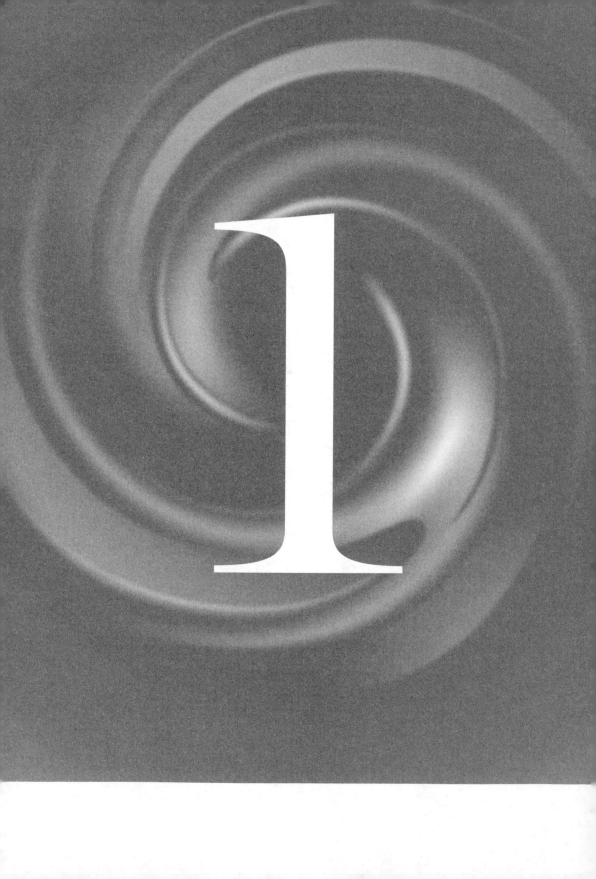

The Rhythm Is Gonna Get You

We are rhythmic beings (our inability to dance notwithstanding), controlled by the beat of the 20,000 nerve cells that make up our body's master clock (tongue-twistingly called the suprachiasmatic nucleus, or as we'll refer to it from here on out, the SCN). This tiny, wing-shaped bit of tissue sits in the hypothalamus in the center of the brain roughly above your ear. For something so small, its power is mighty: Its network of several thousand nerve cells produces a signal that maintains our bodies' 24-hour schedule. In fact, chronobiologists from the University of Murcia in Spain described the SCN as the "conductor of your internal 'orchestra,'" with the musicians being all of your cells and organs.

How all this works is pretty incredible: Light enters your eyes (even when they're closed), kick-starting a process that allows the SCN to sync itself to environmental cues, such as air temperature, food availability, and physical activity. When these rhythm synchers, also called zeitgebers, occur on a more or less regular schedule, all is well.

But when you don't get your light cues at the appropriate times (think blasting your eyes with light from your iPhone at 11:00 p.m. or working in a dark cubicle during daylight hours), or your environmental cues go off schedule (you skip breakfast one morning, and have a Denny's Grand Slam the next), you knock your SCN off its rocker.

What we now call a normal life—frenetic pace, a lack of a structured schedule, staying in darker, inside settings all day while keeping lights on all night—is *not* normal for the SCN. In fact, researchers have a name for the "new normal" that our 21st-century lives have imposed on our circadian rhythms: social jet lag.

The physical result of this new normal? For starters, weight gain.

Why You're Out of Sync

When it comes to your inner clock—actually, clocks, since your body contains tons of them—it's a challenge to visualize the miracle of timing that is happening on a cellular level in your body. Incredibly, every single cell within the SCN contains its own clock, and each cell synchronizes its beat with that of its neighbor cells. Think of one of those desktop toys with the swinging silver balls—you set one in motion, and they all begin to move at the same beat. Our internal beat is maintained by clock genes that produce proteins, which in turn help set off the vibrations that create our circadian rhythms.

WE'VE GOT RHYTHMS

Your body is an amazingly rhythmic creation, a symphony's worth of different rhythms and patterns. And each one plays a role in your health, weight loss, and how you feel every day. Here are some helpful definitions:

CIRCADIAN RHYTHM is your body's 24-hour cycle. (The word *circadian* comes from the Latin *circa dia,* meaning "about a day.") It's well known for affecting your sleep habits, but as you'll find out in this book, it also has a major influence on hunger hormonal secretion and even some activities, such as eating. In addition, circadian rhythms control your sleep/wake cycle, body temperature, blood pressure, reaction time, alertness, and digestion—all of which can impact your weight.

DIURNAL RHYTHMS, again, from *dia,* Latin for day, refer to humans' "standard" circadian rhythm pattern: awake during the day and asleep at night. Many animals, of course—and some people—are nocturnal creatures, sleeping during the day and awake at night. Screw around with your diurnal rhythm too much, and your body won't be able to figure out night from day.

ULTRADIAN RHYTHMS are mini-cycles shorter than 24 hours. The various stages of sleep each night that last 90 to 120 minutes are ultradians. Mealtimes, for example, are also ultradian rhythms: You tend to eat at the same times each day. You have the power to develop certain ultradian rhythms yourself, and they can work for or against your desire to lose weight. Let's say that you take a coffee break every day at 10:30 a.m. and grab a Danish from the snack room. After repeating this for a few days, your body reads this as an ultradian rhythm and begins to expect—that is, crave—that Danish each morning at 10:30.

INFRADIAN RHYTHMS occur in cycles longer than 24 hours. In women, the menstrual cycle is an infradian rhythm; elsewhere in the animal kingdom, hibernation and migration are also examples of infradian rhythms.

Two different vibrations (the science guys call them oscillators) bang out the inner drumbeat we march to when it comes to eating and sleeping. One, called the food-entrained oscillator, or FEO, is cued by—you guessed it—food. The other, the light-entrained oscillator, or LEO, is cued by the daily cycle of light and dark. When the cues for both are in sync, bingo, you do a variety of functions such as eating and sleeping based simply on when you're hungry and tired, in other words, when your body needs them.

But when they're out of sync—which, truth be told, is the perpetual state most of us dwell in these days—they lose their ability to keep you on a natural schedule. And one of the drawbacks is that you're more susceptible to cave in to the urge to eat *even when you're not actually hungry.*

Let's look at each oscillator individually. The FEO is cued by food: It sees food, it wants food. That was okay back in famine times when we weren't sure whether we would get another meal. But now? Not so much. Food is available 24/7, and you see it everywhere—on TV, billboards, in the break room—so your FEO is on continuous overload. This part of our systems has yet to evolve and figure out that there will be a next meal (and a snack, and a dessert), so it's constantly churning out hormones to make you think you're hungry. The FEO's purpose, which worked so well for our hunter-gatherer ancestors, hasn't caught up to modern times.

Then we have the LEO. Again, back in the day when the sunrise told us it was time to get up and sundown told us it was time to go to bed, all was well with this oscillator. But now many of us work out of the sun's glare all day and then fixate in front of artificial light at night, so the LEO is out of whack, too. It keeps you up when you should be sleeping and makes you tired when you should be awake, and it also has lost all sense of when you should eat based on a day/night pattern.

"Our physiology is the same as it was 50,000 years ago, and so is our 'hardware,'" says circadian rhythm expert Akhilesh Reddy, MD, PhD, group leader of the department of clinical neurosciences at the University of Cambridge in England. He notes that this ancient wiring makes it difficult to figure out when we're really hungry and when we should go to bed. "From an evolutionary perspective, at first light we'd go hunting, and then we'd eat. When it got dark, we'd sleep." And how does this affect your weight? If your body doesn't know it's time to sleep, it also doesn't know you shouldn't be eating. "We're more likely to gain weight when we eat food at night because we're meant to metabolize food during daylight hours," says Dr. Reddy.

When Rhythms Go Wrong

It turns out that your natural rhythms are balanced as delicately as a ballerina on her toe shoes. It doesn't take much to throw them off and short-circuit your internal chemistry. When this happens time and time again, you're primed to gain weight—what's more, you also up your risks for chronic diseases and mood swings. Here, some of the key rhythm annihilators:

Sleep deprivation. In their 2010 review of chronobiology studies, a trio of researchers at the University of Murcia in Spain pointed out that women who get 5 hours of sleep a night or fewer weigh nearly 7 pounds more than women who sleep 7 hours. And when University of Chicago researchers restricted a group of healthy young men to 4 hours of sleep nightly for 6 days, they discovered that sleep deprivation impaired glucose tolerance, a precursor of diabetes.

Random eating. We're meant to eat meals on a regular schedule, and doing so trains our bodies to get hungry only at mealtimes. Parents who have put their babies on feeding schedules know this—and revolve their lives around it (a survival skill you'll soon learn will be crucial to lose the weight you want). Eating at random times, meaning not on a set schedule, say researchers, contributes to circadian rhythm disruptions that can affect your health. For example, someone who wakes up late, skips breakfast, and has a late dinner is more likely to have high blood sugar during the night, noted the University of Murcia researchers.

Nighttime eating. People who regularly get the midnight munchies, which researchers call nighttime eating syndrome, or NES, are more than four times more likely to be overweight or obese than people who don't eat at night. It's easy to see why: Nighttime eaters tend to consume almost twice as many carbs as they do during the day.

Shift work. If you're a nurse, a cop, a worker on the night shift, or anyone who works at night and sleeps by day, studies suggest that you're more likely to become obese than your day worker counterparts. What's more, markers of chronic disease occur more often in shift workers than in day workers, and this could trigger metabolic syndrome, say researchers. Metabolic syndrome is a cluster of conditions that include high blood pressure, belly fat, cholesterol imbalances, and glucose intolerance, among other issues. In addition, people with metabolic syndrome are more likely to have heart disease and type 2 diabetes.

All About Belly Fat

There are two different kinds of belly fat, and the Belly Melt Diet's Body Clock Reset will prime you to demolish both. The first kind that you're probably more familiar with is called subcutaneous fat. Subcutaneous fat is the visible flab that pads your thighs and butt, makes your upper arms jiggly, and, er, *fleshes out* your love handles and that spare tire around your middle. The Body Clock Reset is designed to help you cut right through that fat so that you'll actually look forward to shopping for clothes again in no time.

But this program works on another level, as well, to reduce a more dangerous and even poisonous kind of fat. Visceral fat isn't obvious to the naked eye—even people who look skinny on the outside can have too much—and in excess, it can be deadly. In small amounts, visceral fat cushions and protects your internal organs. But just like subcutaneous fat, too much is definitely a bad thing. Smothering the heart, liver, kidneys, and other vital organs with these hormone-pumping fat cells leads to an increased risk of metabolic syndrome (the trifecta of obesity, heart disease, and diabetes), not to mention dementia, cancer, and premature death. It sounds dramatic, but there's good news: Simple lifestyle changes—getting enough sleep, eating the right foods, and getting regular exercise—can radically cut down your visceral fat and add years to your life. Listen closely, dear reader, because throughout the next few chapters, we'll explain why syncing your circadian rhythm and other innate cycles is a surefire way to lose weight and melt your belly fat for good.

Are You Yawning While Reading This?

The number one killer of a healthy circadian rhythm is lack of sleep. And if you're like most Americans, you're exhausted right now. "I'm concerned that we're becoming a sleep-deprived society," says Shawn Youngstedt, PhD, associate professor in the department of exercise science at the University of South Carolina in Columbia. "We sleep an hour less than we did 30 or 40 years ago." And in terms of health, a sleep-deprived society is a sick society.

In fact, recent surveys suggest that we're becoming a nation of "short sleepers." In 2010, University of Chicago researchers published a major survey in the medical journal *Sleep*. In this landmark study, they noted that nearly 1 in 10 people get fewer than 6 hours of sleep a night. And in 2011, a survey of 74,571 people conducted by the Centers for Disease Control and Prevention found that 50 to 70 million American adults "have chronic sleep and wakefulness disorders." Some more numbers to wake you up:

- 35 percent sleep fewer than 7 hours a night (the CDC recommends a minimum of 7 hours a night)
- 48 percent reported that they snored
- 38 percent fell asleep during the day at least once during the previous month
- 4.7 percent reported nodding off while driving in the previous month

If you think yawning all day is the only by-product of a lack of decent shut-eye, think again. The report zeroed in on the harm that a lack of sleep causes: chronic diseases (diabetes and heart disease, for example), mental disorders, health-risk behaviors (smoking and overeating), problems with daily function (that would include falling asleep at your computer), injury, and even death (car accidents caused by sleep-deprived drivers).

All of this, of course, begs the question: Why does too-little sleep lead to weight gain, chronic diseases, and other health problems? A big part of the answer is linked to your hormones, which are cued by light and sleep and, yes, are working on a natural cycle.

Hunger and Hormones (and We Don't Mean the Ones You Usually Hear About)

Just as you have a particular rhythm, your hormones also have a particular rhythm. Hormones (from the Greek word for "impetus") are chemicals secreted by the endocrine glands; they have specific effects on various tissues in your body. In this case, we're not talking about estrogen, progesterone, and testosterone, which are the names women usually associate with hormones (although we'll have more on those later).

No, we're talking about hormones that influence your appetite, aspects of your metabolism, and your sleep/wake cycle. Lack of sleep, which stresses your body, can upend the way these hormones are supposed to work.

It used to be thought that chronic tiredness encouraged weight gain because you were too spent to make healthful meals or head to the gym—and while that's true, research has shown that there's much more to it than simple fatigue. For example, a lack of sleep raises levels of ghrelin, the hormone that triggers the hunger sensation. Less sleep equals a hungrier you—case closed.

Brushing up on how these hormones operate can help you work with them, not against them, and help empower your success with the Belly Melt Diet plan. Here's your hormone cheat sheet.

Cortisol, the stress hormone, is responsible for selecting the carbs, fats, and proteins needed to feed your body's physical demands. Under normal conditions, your adrenal glands release peak levels of cortisol into your blood in the morning to help you wake up; levels taper off in the afternoon and evening. Under stress, cortisol relocates body fat to the fat cell deposits deep inside the abdomen. Can you say, "Bring on the belly fat"?

Ghrelin, the hunger hormone, originates in the stomach. Levels of this hunger-making chemical rise before mealtime and drop after you eat. Basically, ghrelin is what tells you it's chow time. And it steers you not only to food but to high-calorie ones. According to a 2010 study by researchers at the Imperial College of London, ghrelin increases the appeal of high-calorie—but not low-calorie—foods.

High levels of ghrelin, which was discovered in 1999, mimic your body's response to fasting by making you feel ravenous (even when your body has enough fuel). Research shows that not getting enough sleep at night actually triggers your body to create more of this ever-hungry hormone.

Leptin, the starvation hormone, is key to the long-term regulation of body weight, and is secreted mostly by fat cells. When at the proper levels, leptin tells you that you're full or that it's not time to eat just yet. Researchers at Rockefeller University in New York City, who discovered leptin in 1994 via experiments on mice, report that it regulates body weight by signaling the amount of fat you store.

While this may sound like a dieter's dream, leptin is also the hormone that can thwart aggressive dieting. Here's how: Your leptin levels are pretty much set at a certain level. At that level or above, your brain senses that you have enough energy on board. So you eat appropriate amounts of food, get enough exercise, and burn energy at a normal rate. But dieting actually decreases the amount of leptin your body produces (fat cells secrete leptin, so fewer fat cells equals less leptin). It's a lack of leptin that researchers believe tells your body that it's starving, when in fact you're only dieting, making you feel even hungrier when you cut back on calories. Another leptin depleter is not enough sleep.

Melatonin, the sleep hormone, regulates other hormones and plays a key role in maintaining your circadian rhythms. Produced in your pineal gland when it's dark out, melatonin production slows as morning dawns. Even a little light can lessen the flow of melatonin at night when you need it most; for instance, being exposed to bright light late in the evening, shift work, jet lag, and even bad vision can lower melatonin levels, as can getting too little light during the day—all of which translates to poor sleep. And here's something you may have missed back in bio class: Melatonin also helps control the release of female hormones; it determines the timing of a girl's first period, the frequency and length of her menstrual cycle, and the onset of menopause.

The takeaway: Lack of sleep can throw off all of these hormones, making you defenseless against another piece of cake; being out of whack, these hormones can also sabotage your weight loss efforts by telling your body to hold on to stubborn belly fat, even when you are being good. Like we said, it's a vicious cycle.

The Other Hormones on the Clock

Melatonin and the hunger hormones aren't the only ones whose levels ebb and flow through your body like the tides. Other hormone levels vary throughout your day and your cycle, too—and, according to a 2010 study published in the *International Journal of Endocrinology,* by Diane B. Boivin, MD, PhD, founder of the Center for Study and Treatment of Circadian Rhythms at the Douglas Institute/McGill University in Montreal, these variations can affect your sleep. When hormonal swells and dips cause bouts of too little sleep, it can set the stage for bouts of another unwelcome activity—overeating.

Estrogen is involved in the flow of melatonin, say researchers, who continue to work on uncovering the estrogen-melatonin connection. This much we do know: Estrogen seems to reduce melatonin's sleep-inducing action, says Robert J. Hedaya, MD, clinical professor of psychiatry at Georgetown University. Especially after ovulation, estrogen can lessen the amount of REM sleep—the important, restful phase marked by rapid eye movements—during which we dream. Without REM sleep, the sleep we get isn't as beneficial.

Progesterone. When you are premenstrual, it's likely that you have lower levels of this hormone. A reproductive hormone that induces sleep, progesterone is also known to have antianxiety effects on sleep, a phenomenon that researchers compare with that of tranquilizers. (Hence, the increased anxiety and reduced sleep during that oh-so-wonderful time of the month.)

It's Not Your Fault

The message of this chapter is this: These stealth cycles, some of which you probably didn't even know about, are running the show in terms of your health and weight. But the frenetic way we live our lives today, combined with the ways in which we often try to lose weight—following rigid diets, going hungry—actually work against these rhythms. Now you understand why being tired has helped you hang on to your weight, and why starving yourself on crazy diets did nothing more than trigger your hormones to go into overdrive and send you right into the arms of a Big Mac. You *can't* fight your body and win.

But here's the good news: You *can* work with these cycles to make weight loss easier. You can harness your body's natural rhythms to steamroll your belly, energize your life, and feel great all the time.

Now that you know about these cycles, the next step is to use them to your advantage. The Belly Melt Diet is broken down into three main components: resetting your body's circadian rhythm, realigning your eating patterns with what your body needs at the right times, and reestablishing your fitness routine to maximize its effectiveness—in other words, work out smarter, not harder. Everything about the program is designed to break the cycle of weight gain by getting your body back in touch with its natural rhythm. Here is an overview of the plan's three main areas.

The Body Clock Reset: If there's been a crucial breakthrough in weight loss research recently, it's how important getting the right amount of sleep is to becoming and staying slim. This section (which you've already started) will help you not only reset your circadian rhythm so that you can sleep better at night but also maximize your energy and control your hunger hormones all day.

The Reset and Reshape Diets: A quick-start 3-day plan will reset your hunger hormones to stop cravings. First, you'll eat at specific times, so the hunger hormones are under control at all times. Second, you'll be eating meals and snacks that provide a perfect balance of carbs, protein, and fats to keep those hormones under control, and that will stimulate you when you need it (during the day) and calm you when you don't (when it's time to go to sleep). Third, you'll be choosing foods with nutrients that will help you sleep better, which in turn will help reset your body clock so the weight will come off faster. Since the plan focuses on whole, nonprocessed foods, you'll not only feel healthier but you'll kick any addictions to refined sugar and additives, which are also messing with your body clock and feeding that toxic visceral fat.

The Perfect-Timing Workout: The best part about the Belly Melt Diet workout is that it isn't hard, it isn't time-consuming—in fact, it's pretty simple. What makes this plan different is that when you do it—by doing cardio and strength training and stretching at certain times of the day—you'll see faster results. And you'll feel better while you're doing it (so you'll stick with it) because you'll be working with your body's rhythms instead of forcing it to move when it doesn't want to (yes, your body has a set of rhythms that control when it wants to exercise). Perfectly timed exercise also helps reset your sleep-wake cycle. And if you say you don't have time, consider this: Each workout is broken down into 20-minute segments that you can fit into any schedule.

In addition to this core plan, throughout the book you'll see recurring boxes called "Hit the Reset Button." These are key tips that have been scientifically proven to help you reset your body clock so that you can lose the weight you want and feel rested. And once you put yourself on a schedule that works in harmony with your internal rhythms, you'll discover, to your delight, that the weight you lose on this program will stay lost—once and for all.

WHAT'S YOUR BEST TIME?

Your body temperature is a great way to figure out what your peak time of day is. Here's how to discover yours: Take your temperature every 2 hours or so for 5 or 6 consecutive days and record it. It's best to do this on a sheet of graph paper. (Try for at least three recordings between midnight and 5:00 a.m. And be sure to stay in bed when you record your nighttime temps.)

In general, your body temperature tends to fluctuate by plus or minus 1.5 degrees throughout the day. Here's what's important: When your temperature begins to rise, you tend to be awake and primed for peak performance. When it ebbs to its lowest level, you feel sleepy. This temperature test can also help larks and owls take advantage of their natural schedule.

LARKS: You'll notice that your temperature peaks at around midnight, then steadily drops until reaching its lowest point around 5:00 a.m. By 6:00 a.m. or so, it stays more or less the same till 8:30. During this time, you can either sleep or rise. If you charted your daily temperature fluctuations, you'd see this time as pretty much a straight line. But starting about 9:00 a.m., a lark's temperature rises steadily, which means you're at your most alert. This is a good time to hunker down and work, for this is when larks tend to be the most productive. By 1:00 p.m. or so, your temperature will "flatline" for a few hours, signaling that it's time for a quick siesta or, failing that, simple tasks that don't need maximum brain power. And from around 4:00 p.m. until 10:00 p.m., your temperature rises steadily again, ushering in another several hours of alertness that drops off later, around 11:00 p.m., as your temperature goes back down. For larks, it's bedtime.

OWLS: You owlish night birds will find that your body temperature peaks between 1:00 a.m. and 3:00 a.m., and then declines rather sharply until reaching a low about 8:00 a.m. From 8:00 a.m. till noon, temps rise, even though you may not. So owls are at their most churlish in the morning, and if they have day jobs, tend to be sluggish and maybe even a little grumpy. Starting about 3:00 p.m., temps flatten out until about 6:00 p.m., and then rise to a high between midnight and 3:00 a.m. So, come late afternoon, owls begin to come alive—most will stay happy and alert until the wee hours.

QUIZ: What Kind of Bird Are You?

Though we're all hardwired by our SCN, we're not all wired the same way, and researchers have come up with terms to help describe each group of people. Some are "larks," who happily get up with the sun and who go to bed every night well before midnight. Others are "owls," night birds who rise between 9:00 a.m. and noon, and may not get to bed till the wee hours.

These predispositions are probably hereditary—linked genetically in ways that researchers are still unraveling. Though many of us have bits of both lark and owl aspects, it's helpful to figure out what your dominant body rhythm is so you can maximize what works best for you. Taking this fun quiz will help you do just that. The number of points for each answer appears in parentheses. When you're done, add up your points and check the key following the quiz to find out what kind of bird you are.

1. How hungry are you first thing in the morning?

a. I can't stand the sight of food. (1)

b. If you make me something, maybe I'll nibble. (2)

c. I'm ready to eat. (3)

d. I'd like the breakfast special with everything, please! (4)

2. What is your energy level like right after you get up?

a. Can't I just stay in bed? (1)

b. I can barely drag myself to the shower. (2)

c. Ah, it's morning—time to get going. (3)

d. I'm heading right out for my morning 5K! (4)

3. It's Friday night. What's your bedtime compared with work nights?

a. It's the same. I'm a creature of habit. (4)

b. I push myself to stay up for *The Daily Show* and some of *The Colbert Report*. (3)

c. I love staying up late on weekend nights—but can only last an hour or two past my usual bedtime. (2)

d. TGIF! I'm going out on the town. (1)

4. You're considering taking an exercise class. There's a convenient one nearby that starts at 7:00 a.m. How will you do?

a. That's a perfect time for me to work out at the max. (4)

b. I expect I won't embarrass myself. (3)

c. I'll stand in the back row so no one sees me. (2)

d. Ugh, this is going to be ugly. (1)

5. At night, when are you most likely to fade to black?

a. 8:00 p.m. to 9:00 p.m. (5)

b. 9:00 p.m. to 10:15 p.m. (4)

c. 10:15 p.m. to 12:45 a.m. (3)

d. 12:45 a.m. to 2:00 a.m. (2)

e. 2:00 a.m. to 3:00 a.m. (1)

6. How does an 11:00 p.m. bedtime make you feel?

a. I'll go, but I'm really not tired. (0)

b. Okay, I could sleep, I guess. (2)

c. Sounds just about right. (3)

d. Exhausted. I should've been in bed an hour ago. (5)

7. If you had to stay awake between 4:00 a.m. and 6:00 a.m., and had an empty schedule all day after that, what would you do?

a. Something entertaining until 4:00 a.m. and go to bed at 6:00 a.m. (1)

b. Take a nap before 4:00 a.m. and again after 6:00 a.m. (2)

c. Go to bed at my normal time, wake up at 4:00 a.m., and nap after 6:00 a.m. (3)

d. Go to bed at my usual time, wake up at 4:00 a.m., and stay awake after 6:00 a.m. (4)

8. At what time of day do you shine?

a. Midnight to 5:00 a.m. (1)

b. 5:00 a.m. to 9:00 a.m. (5)

c. 9:00 a.m. to 11:00 a.m. (4)

d. 11:00 a.m. to 5:00 p.m. (3)

e. 5:00 p.m. to 10:00 p.m. (2)

f. 10:00 p.m. to midnight (1)

9. Which are you, a lark or an owl?

a. Definitely a lark. I wake up singing! (6)

b. I'm up with the birds; I must be a lark. (4)

c. A little more owl than lark—what kind of bird does that make me? (2)

d. Hooot! Hooooot! (0)

10. You get to choose your work hours—what time do you start your day?

a. Midnight to 3:00 a.m. (1)

b. 3:00 a.m. to 8:00 a.m. (5)

c. 8:00 a.m. to 10:00 a.m. (4)

d. 10:00 a.m. to 2:00 p.m. (3)

e. 2:00 p.m. to 4:00 p.m. (2)

f. 4:00 p.m. to midnight (1)

11. Lucky you! You won the lottery and have taken a permanent vacation. You can do whatever you like, whenever. When do you go to bed?

a. 8:00 p.m. to 9:00 p.m. (6)

b. 9:00 p.m. to 10:00 p.m. (5)

c. 10:00 p.m. to 11:00 p.m. (4)

d. 11:00 p.m. to midnight (3)

e. Midnight to 1:00 a.m. (2)

f. 1:00 a.m. to 2:30 a.m. (1)

g. After 2:30 a.m. (0)

12. You're still on permanent vacation, you lucky human. When is it your pleasure to wake up?

a. Anytime before 6:00 a.m. (6)

b. 6:00 a.m. to 7:00 a.m. (5)

c. 7:00 a.m. to 8:00 a.m. (4)

d. 8:00 a.m. to 9:00 a.m. (3)

e. 9:00 a.m. to 10:30 a.m. (2)

f. 10:30 a.m. to noon (1)

g. After noon (0)

---

8 to 20 points: No doubt about it, you're a creature of the night.

21 to 30 points: You prefer sleeping in and staying up late.

31 to 45 points: You prefer the day but like the occasional late night.

46 to 58 points: You're up with the sun, and 11:00 p.m. is late for you.

Why this matters: Larks may have an easier time resetting their clocks' natural rhythms. But owls, forced to go at it in this 9-to-5 world, may feel exhausted and out of step most of the time. See Chapter 3 for tricks that will help you reset your clock.

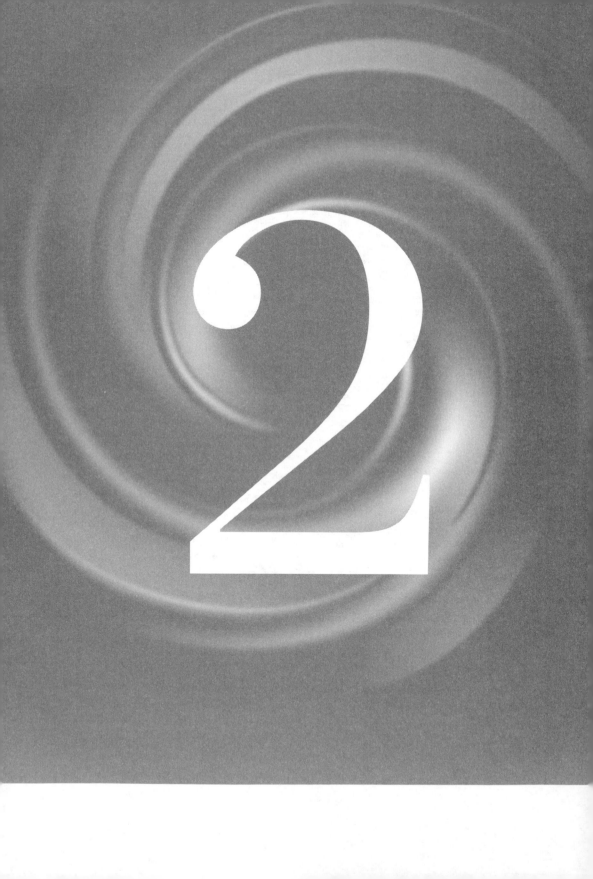

Sleep Yourself Thin

Most diet programs center around the kitchen—whether your own or a restaurant's. While it makes sense, in theory, to focus on what you eat as a source of weight loss or gain, there's another room in your house that may be much more important in the battle against stubborn belly fat, as major breakthroughs in weight loss research have shown in the past few years. And that room is where you should spend at least 7 to 9 hours each night.

Yes, your bedroom is key to the Belly Melt Diet program. Believe it or not, sleeping is one of the most powerful weight loss tools ever discovered. As you'll read below, quality shut-eye—and the subsequent benefits on your internal circadian rhythm—plays a major role in how your body registers hunger and satiety. Plus, resetting your sleep clock will help increase your energy—giving you even more of what you need to lose the weight.

And unlike other weight loss programs, pills, and potions you've probably tried over the years, there are no negative side effects. Sleeping right will not only help you lose weight but will also help prevent a slew of chronic diseases and mood disorders. And unlike pills, proper sleep really works as a weight loss tool, and it has an unparalleled safety record. Yet, despite its safety record, effectiveness, and wonderful side benefits, we're willing to bet that your doctor has never once prescribed it for weight loss.

All that stands between you and the weight loss you want is a solid 7 to 9 hours of deep sleep every night. Here's what you need to know about how sleep can help you defeat the battle of your belly (and thigh and butt) fat.

The Weight Battle of the Short Sleeper

If you're what researchers call a short sleeper (measured not by height but by how long you sleep each night—5.5 to 6 hours or less qualifies you), you'll have trouble losing weight, no doubt about it. In a 7-year study of 7,022 middle-aged people, Finnish researchers found that women who reported sleep problems were more likely to experience a major weight gain (defined as 11 pounds or more).

You know that sleep and weight gain may be linked, but why is that? Here's what the earth-shattering new research has revealed, and why lack of sleep could be stalling your ability to lose weight and keep it off:

Sleep less, burn less. In a study at the department of neuroendocrinology at the University of Lübeck, Germany, published in the *American Journal of Clinical Nutrition,* researchers had a group of men sleep for 12 hours a night but didn't allow them to sleep the next night, and then had them eat an opulent buffet the following morning. Then the researchers measured the subjects' energy expenditure—the calories you burn just by being. When the men were sleep-deprived, their general energy expenditure was 5 percent less than it was when they got a good night's sleep, and their post-meal energy expenditure was 20 percent less.

Sleep less, eat more. In research presented at the American Heart Association's 2011 Scientific Sessions, it was shown that women who got only 4 hours of sleep at night ate 329 additional calories the next day than they did after they slept 9 hours. (Men ate 263 calories more.) In another study published in the *American Journal of Clinical Nutrition,* 11 volunteers spent 14 days at a sleep center on two occasions. During one period, they slept 5.5 hours a night, and during the other, they slept 8.5 hours. When the subjects were sleep-deprived, they increased their nighttime snacking and were more likely to choose high-carbohydrate snacks.

Sleep less, crave more. This is probably the biggest revelation about the connection between sleep and weight loss—and the biggest challenge for you if you're not getting at least 7 solid hours of sleep each night. Sleeping too little impacts your hormone levels in ways that can undermine the efforts of even the most determined dieter. That's because insufficient sleep raises the levels of ghrelin, the hormone that tells you to eat. When it comes to weight gain and loss, this hormone plays a leading role.

Ghrelin's job is to boost your appetite, increase fat production, and make your body grow—all of which are fine things if you're a lanky 12-year-old. But once you're in your thirties, ghrelin's effects can seem pretty darned undesirable. It's a cinch to figure out why this hormone is the last thing a dieter needs to have circulating in excess.

Lack of sleep also lowers levels of leptin, the hormone that says, "I'm full; put the fork down." And leptin has a circadian rhythm all its own: Leptin's levels run high during the night, which tells your body while you're

THE HEALTHY SIDE OF SLEEP

You deal with the fallout of not getting enough sleep by feeling a little groggy every morning. But what you may not realize is the domino effect at work here, and it's much more insidious than just feeling tired. Increasingly, researchers tell us, it's clear that "short sleeping" can get us into plenty of trouble healthwise. Insufficient sleep is linked not only to obesity—which brings its own set of health issues—but also to a host of other maladies. Here's a sampling:

CARDIOVASCULAR DISEASE. In a 2010 study published in the journal *Sleep,* researchers at the West Virginia University School of Medicine reviewed data from 30,397 people who had participated in the 2005 National Health Interview Study. They discovered that those sleeping fewer than 7 hours a night were at increased risk of heart disease. In particular, women under 60 who sleep 5 hours or fewer a night have twice the risk for developing heart disease.

DIABETES. According to a study in the journal *Diabetes* in 2011, University of Chicago and Northwestern University researchers found that when people with type 2 diabetes slept poorly at night, they had a 9 percent higher fasting glucose level, a 30 percent higher fasting insulin level, and a 43 percent higher insulin resistance level. Diabetics with insomnia fared even worse—their fasting glucose levels were 23 percent higher, their fasting insulin levels were 48 percent higher, and their insulin resistance levels were 82 percent higher than diabetics who didn't have insomnia.

BREAST CANCER. Researchers at Tohoku University Graduate School of Medicine in Sendai, Japan, studied data from nearly 24,000 women ages 40 to 79, and learned that those who slept fewer than 6 hours a night had a

sleeping that you don't need to eat. Its levels drop during the day, when you need food as energy. So high leptin levels keep hunger at bay. In studies, for example, mice lost weight because leptin made them eat less and exercise more: the holy grail of dieting. But if you don't get enough sleep, your leptin levels plummet.

So after even one night of too little sleep, leptin and ghrelin become dietary gremlins bent on diet-wrecking mischief. The lower leptin levels mean that you still feel hungry after you eat. And ghrelin, for its part, magnifies the

62 percent higher risk for breast cancer, while those who slept more than 9 hours a night had a 28 percent lower risk.

COLON CANCER. In a study of 1,240 people published in 2011, Case Western University researchers found that those who slept fewer than 6 hours a night were 47 percent more likely to have colorectal polyps, which can become cancerous, than people who clocked at least 7 hours of sleep.

URINARY PROBLEMS. In findings presented at the May 2011 meeting of the American Urological Association, researchers at the New England Research Institute in Watertown, Massachusetts, reviewed data from 4,145 middle-aged men and women and here's what they discovered: Five years of sleeping restlessly or too little (fewer than 5 hours a night) can increase by 80 to 90 percent a woman's risk of needing to wake at night to urinate (nocturia) or of becoming incontinent. A whopping 42 percent of the women classified themselves as restless sleepers, compared with 34 percent of the men. The researchers theorize that sleeping poorly causes inflammation, which in turn can lead to urinary problems.

MORTALITY. A 10-year study of some 16,000 people by researchers at the University of Copenhagen connected the dots between a lack of sleep and an increased risk of mortality. It turns out that the men who reported sleeping badly, especially those under 45, had twice the risk for death than men who reported sleeping well. And men who had three or more sleep disturbances a night had a suicide risk five times higher than men whose sleep was undisturbed. Though sleep disturbances didn't affect women's mortality, both women and men who reported sleep disturbances were more likely to have high blood pressure and diabetes.

problem by stimulating your appetite, setting the stage for a day of unsatisfying, high-cal feasting after a restless night.

In the Wisconsin Sleep Cohort Study of more than 1,000 people, researchers found that people who got 5 hours of sleep a night had 15.5 percent lower leptin levels and 14.9 percent higher levels of ghrelin, compared with those who got 8 hours of sleep. Know what else the nonsleepers scored higher numbers in? BMI. So more ghrelin plus less leptin equals greater body mass index *and* weight gain.

In a study at the University of Chicago, researchers discovered that restricting the sleep of 12 healthy young men to 4 hours a night lowered their leptin levels by 18 percent. The men rated themselves as having a 24 percent increase in hunger.

Sleep less, hang on to fat more. Lack of sleep may also affect the *kind* of weight you lose. In another study at the University of Chicago, researchers followed 10 overweight but healthy subjects who were placed on a balanced diet, then observed in two 14-day increments, one in which they got about 7.5 hours of sleep, and another in which they got 5 hours and 15 minutes. During both periods, the subjects lost an average of 6.6 pounds. But when they got more sleep, they lost 3.1 pounds of fat, whereas during the short-sleep period, they lost only 1.3 pounds of fat. Those who got more sleep reported less hunger, which makes sense: When they got enough sleep, their ghrelin levels stayed the same. On the 5-hour nights, their ghrelin levels rose by 9 points.

Since ghrelin also promotes the retention of fat, researchers theorize that a lack of sleep explains why the nonsleepers held on to body fat. This happens because the diet-unfriendly hormone reduces the number of calories you burn off and increases glucose production.

Sleep less, have more time to eat. It hasn't been scientifically proven, but some experts believe that the 2 hours or more that we're no longer using to sleep is giving us another 2 hours to raid the fridge.

The Sleep/Belly Fat Connection

Here's something else we bet you didn't know. When you gain weight as fat, you're enlarging more than your waistline. You're actually enlarging the size of fat tissues that have their own circadian rhythm and secrete their own hormones and other chemicals—some of which have decidedly unhealthful effects.

Back in 1994, when researchers at Rockefeller University in New York City discovered the hormone leptin, they sparked a revolution in the way we study and understand obesity. With this discovery came the revelation that body fat isn't just gobs of inert blobs that bump out your belly and enlarge your nether regions. They found that fat acts almost as a pseudo gland, in that it releases substances on its own.

And as you read in the previous studies, a lack of sleep produces more ghrelin, which tells your body to "hold on tight to those fat cells!" So the less sleep you get, the more your body hangs on to fat and the more those sleepy fat cells churn out either too much or too little of the following substances. Here's a primer:

TNF. You would think this was something you'd want around—it kills tumor cells. But as with so many things, a little is good, but a lot is overkill. This protein promotes inflammation (linked to diseases including heart disease, diabetes, arthritis, and cancer).

YOU DO NEED YOUR BEAUTY SLEEP

As if you needed scientific proof that you don't look so hot after not getting enough sleep, a group of Dutch researchers did a study on the effects of sleep (and the lack of it) on beauty. In a study published in the *British Medical Journal,* the research-ers took photos of 23 healthy people after they'd had a good night's sleep—and then photographed them after they'd been awake for 31 hours.

Later, they showed the photos to 65 random people, who rated the snapshots as to the subject's health, attractiveness, and tiredness. Lending weight to the notion that getting your beauty sleep really pays off, the observers ranked the people who didn't sleep as looking more tired, less healthy, and—wait for it—less attractive than those who'd gotten a full night's sleep.

Quick take: Sleep deprivation increases disease-promoting TNF levels.

Adiponectin. Only fat cells produce and secrete this hormone, which fights inflammation and helps protect against heart disease. A recent Harvard Medical School study discovered the connection between it and sleep loss, finding that, among Caucasian women, sleep deprivation produced lower levels of this health-promoting hormone.

Quick take: This may explain why women who don't get enough sleep are at higher risk for heart attacks.

Visfatin. High levels of this fat-produced chemical messenger affect insulin resistance and seem to play a role in inflammatory gut problems such as Crohn's disease and ulcerative colitis.

Quick take: Sleep deprivation increases levels of visfatin.

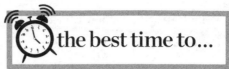

the best time to...

HAVE SURGERY

In the morning, and not just because you get it over with sooner. A 2006 study at Duke University that looked at 90,000 operations found that patients who were operated on before noon experienced less pain and nausea and fewer complications. The low came with surgeries that began at 9:00 a.m., when 1 percent of patients experienced these adverse effects, compared with 4.2 percent of patients who were operated on at 4:00 p.m. Researchers say circadian rhythms are probably at play, with surgeons and patients alike experiencing an afternoon dip in alertness and energy.

Make Time to Sleep

By now you've surely connected the dots between poor sleep and those extra inches around your belly and thighs. In the next chapter, we'll address the ways to get a good night's sleep, night after night.

But perhaps your problem isn't that you can't sleep—it's that you just don't have the time to sleep. We just can't say this strongly enough: If you

DOES SLEEPLESSNESS MAKE YOU EVIL?

Well, not evil exactly, but it could render you ruder, more apt to respond inappropriately—and might even make you an unethical money grubber, say researchers from the University of North Carolina and the University of Arizona. In their study of sleep-deprived students, the researchers found that pulling an all-nighter led to increased "deviant and unethical" behavior. According to the researchers, a lack of sleep affects brain function in the prefrontal cortex, which in turn controls behavior.

don't get 7 or 8 hours' worth of uninterrupted sleep at night, you're going to be much less likely to lose weight. Or you'll lose a quick 10 to 20 pounds, only to gain it back within a year or two. And weight issues won't be your only problem if you consistently get fewer than 6 hours of sleep a night: This puts you squarely in the danger zone for diabetes, heart disease, and breast and colon cancer.

As for not having time to sleep, we understand that women today are pushed and pulled from every angle, and sometimes it seems like the only time to get things done is after *Letterman* or before the rooster crows.

Our first argument is that you're worth the commitment. A better night's sleep not only will make for a skinner and healthier you but for a more energetic you—and a more energetic you can get a lot more things done. Giving up sleep to check off another item on your to-do list really is a case of diminishing returns—you're so tired that there's no way you're doing things effectively or efficiently.

We'd also like to say: You probably *do* have the time. For the next 2 weeks, we want you to keep a time diary. Log your days in 15-minute increments. At the end of the 2 weeks, we bet you'll find that you've engaged

EXERCISE YOUR ZZZ'S

For years, many people—including experts—thought that exercising in the evening revs you up and keeps you awake. Well, put that myth to rest, says Shawn Youngstedt, PhD, associate professor in the department of exercise science at the University of South Carolina in Columbia, who has been studying sleep and exercise for 2 decades. "It makes intuitive sense that late exercise impairs sleep, but it's not true," Dr. Youngstedt says. "Large surveys show that people who exercise at night sleep better."

A study published by the Japanese Society of Sleep Research confirms this and adds another benefit: daytime alertness. Researchers had the study's subjects exercise at different times of day, and then monitored their sleep. When they exercised in the evening, the subjects not only slept better at night but they also reported feeling less sleepy during the day. Researchers concluded that wakefulness during the day promotes restful slow-wave (deep) sleep in the first sleep cycle of the night. In effect, late-day exercise kicks off a cycle of restful nights and wide-awake days. Another study, done by Finnish researchers and published in the *Journal of Sleep Research* in 2011, found that even vigorous late-night exercise did not affect the quality of the subjects' sleep.

When you stop to think about it, exercising *should* make you sleep better. After working out, your body is tired and ready for rest. Furthermore, what happens after exercise mimics bodily changes that prepare you for sleep: your heart rate, blood pressure, and body temperature all trend downward. So if the only time you can work out is in the evening, don't worry that it's too close to bedtime. (In fact, as you'll read in Chapter 10, it's the best time to work out in terms of maximizing your fat burn and building lean muscle.)

Of course, if you find that late-night exercise is messing with your sleep, you should go with the timing that works for you. "It's not the case for most people, but there are some for whom exercise within 2 hours of bedtime impairs sleep," notes Dr. Youngstedt. If you're one of them, chalk it up to being an outlier in his research, and move your workout up a little earlier in the day; 3 hours before bedtime should be a good margin. It's all about finding the right daily rhythm for you.

in activities that aren't nearly as healthful for you as an extra couple of hours' sleep at night are.

Take watching TV, for example. According to a 2009 article in the *New York Times,* here's the average amount of time Americans spent watching television per day during the 2008–2009 season:

Age Range	Hours
65+	6:41
50–64	5:52
35–49	4:55
18–34	4:10

By this time, it should be clear that replacing just 2 hours of watching TV with 2 hours of sleep is one of the best investments you can make for your health. And if you need a little more convincing, check out this widely reported 2011 study of 4,512 Scottish adults, published in the *Journal of the American College of Cardiology.* Its findings? That people who spend 2 or more hours a day in front of a screen are far more likely to die of any cause and to suffer heart-related problems than those who don't watch the boob tube as much, according to researchers from University College in London. Compared with people who spend fewer than 2 hours a day on screen-based entertainment (watching TV, using a computer, or playing video games), those who had more screen time experienced a 48 percent increase in death from all causes and a 125 percent increase in cardiovascular events—even once the researchers factored in variables like smoking, high blood pressure, weight, and exercise.

So as you can see, if you make the time (and you probably have the time already), you'll see benefits everywhere—your energy levels, your dress size, and your outlook on life.

OHM YOURSELF TO SLEEP

Yoga breathing is designed to relax the body and quiet the mind, so it's no surprise that it can soothe us toward sleep. Sleep specialist Phillip Eichling, MD, director of the Comprehensive Sleep Solutions lab in Tucson and a medical director of Canyon Ranch, recommends Zen breath watching. Taking slow, deep breaths while counting each one, 1 to 10, over and over (repeating the numbers rather than counting higher avoids agitating yourself by thinking, "I'm at 123 already; why aren't I asleep?") can get you to sleep at bedtime or back to sleep if you wake up later on.

Just before bed, the right movements can prepare your body to drift off. Studies have shown that yoga can help you fall asleep faster, go back to sleep after middle-of-the-night awakenings, and have a longer, more restful sleep. A study at the division of sleep medicine at Harvard Medical School found that yoga signifi-cantly improved the ability of people with insomnia to fall asleep and stay asleep. Making 5 minutes of yoga part of your routine before bed each night can help direct the sandman your way. Whichever asanas you choose, hold them for a minute or more, breathing deeply. Try the following poses that are restorative rather than energizing (for more yoga moves, see page 313):

LEGS-UP-THE-WALL INVERSION. Lie on the floor with your butt against a wall and your legs raised 90 degrees, resting them against the wall.

Sleep Off the Pounds

At this point you should be sold on the idea that sleeping is a major part of effective weight loss—and a focal point of the Belly Melt Diet program. Just think about it: You're on a diet, exercising, and doing all the right things, but like most Americans, you shortchange yourself in the sleep department. Thanks to a lack of shut-eye, your body is churning out ghrelin, making you hungry. It's also shutting down leptin, the hormone that signals your body to stop eating. That's why you can't resist the doughnuts in the break room or an extra serving of fries at dinner—not because you lack *willpower* but because you lack *sleep.*

SEATED FORWARD BEND. Sit on the floor with your legs extended in front of you, and bend over them, grasping your calves or toes. The point here is to stretch and relax, so don't grunt or pull to admire how flexible you are.

CHILD'S POSE. Resting your tush on your heels, lean forward until your head is resting on the floor. If it doesn't, support your head with a pillow. Your arms can be extended forward on either side of your head or back along your sides, the way a baby sleeps.

PLOW. Some yoga experts also recommend an inversion such as the plow before bed, as long as it's not strenuous: Lie on your back, raise your legs over your head, and bring them down behind your head. Your toes can touch the floor if you're flexible enough, or you can rest them on a pillow.

SAVASANA. This simple—but amazingly profound—yoga pose is often called the corpse pose because "it's a little like playing dead," says Amy Wechsler, MD, adjunct assistant clinical professor of psychiatry at Weill Cornell Medical College in New York City. Dr. Wechsler says this pose can help you relax completely before bedtime. Here's how to do it: Lie on your back on a cushioned surface, arms at your sides, not touching your body, palms up. Slowly sink into the pose, breathing naturally, and letting your body go limp. Stay in this position for a few minutes or as long as you like.

Even if you can fight through these food desires, the extra ghrelin kicked up because of those sleepless nights is holding on for dear life to every fat cell you have. This disruption of your body's circadian rhythm, combined with other natural cycle killers (see Chapter 1 for a reminder), sets you up for a sequence of cravings, hunger, and frustration—all of which make losing weight a virtual impossibility.

Now that you know you need a good night's sleep to melt your belly fat, the next chapters will tell you just how to do it.

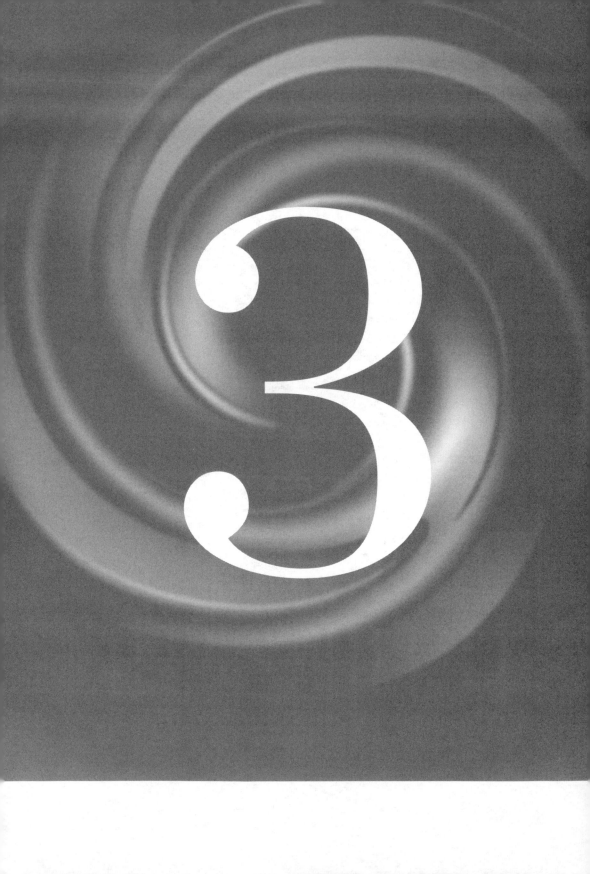

Get the Sleep of Your Dreams

Once you realize that your success at following the Belly Melt Diet depends on getting a good night's sleep, you may be thinking, "Okay, great—now what? I don't sleep like a baby, and I have no idea how to turn things around. Where do I start?"

Start with this fun quiz, the BMD Sleepy Scale, which is based on tests used by sleep experts. Your score will let you know whether or not you're getting enough restful sleep.

1. When your alarm goes off at 7:00 a.m., what's your reaction?
    a. Alarm? Alarms are for sissies! I'm up by 7:00 and raring to go.
    b. I curse silently, then turn off the alarm and get out of bed.
    c. When I say I hit the snooze button, I mean I *really* hit it.
    d. This. Cannot. Be. Happening. To. Me.

2. You're on your way to work. How are you doing?
    a. Just fine, thanks. How are *you* doin'?
    b. I'm on autopilot. Will reach destination on time.
    c. Moving very slowly today. Is there coffee?
    d. Doing the slow crawl to the office.

3. Your honey suggests a romantic night. You:
    a. Get out the candles and your sexiest nightie.
    b. Hope for a quickie.
    c. Wonder if he'll notice that you're on snooze control.
    d. Ask for a rain check.

4. It's your book club night. You:
    a. Organize notes on Post-its so you won't forget a thing.
    b. Chime in with a pithy comment now and then.
    c. Look thoughtful and try to nod in the right places.
    d. Fall asleep on the couch.

5. At night, how many hours do you usually sleep?
    a. 8 to 9.
    b. 7 to 8.
    c. 6 to 7.
    d. Less than 6.

6. It's finally Friday. What time will you get up tomorrow?
    a. My usual, of course—7:00 a.m.
    b. I'll be up by 8:00 or so.
    c. See you at 9-ish.
    d. Don't call me before noon.

7. You're watching a *Law & Order* rerun. You . . .

    a. Watch till the very end, even though you know who done it.

    b. Pay attention until they hit the courtroom.

    c. Start dosing off during the autopsy.

    d. Don't make it past the opening credits and fall asleep on the couch.

8. On a free afternoon, what are the chances that you'll catch a nap?

    a. Not a chance! I don't nap—I *do stuff.*

    b. I might sit quietly and read, but I rarely fall asleep.

    c. There's a pretty good chance that I'll close my eyes.

    d. I'm napping just thinking about a free afternoon.

9. Once in bed, you . . .

    a. Relax with a good book for a bit, then fall right asleep.

    b. Hope you'll fall asleep quickly, and you usually do.

    c. Fall asleep, then wake up 2 hours later, and toss and turn the rest of the night.

    d. Stare at the ceiling all night.

10. What's your eating and exercise schedule like?

    a. Three meals a day, every day. And I walk 30 minutes a day.

    b. I'm more or less regular about both.

    c. I eat.

    d. What was the question?

Key:

Mostly A answers: Good news! If these answers are typical of you over time, chances are that you're getting enough sleep. You can skip ahead to the diet and exercise parts of the Belly Melt Diet.

Mostly B answers: You're doing pretty well in the sleep department but still need to pay attention to our suggestions for relaxation.

Mostly C answers: You're not a good sleeper, but you probably already know that. The suggestions in this chapter will help you learn how to get a good night's rest.

Mostly D answers: You may have a sleep disorder. Pay your doctor a visit to rule out physical problems such as sleep apnea, and strictly follow the suggestions in this chapter.

Why Can't I Sleep?

It seems so simple: Hit the pillow, sleep, get up. But for millions of Americans, that scenario is just a dream. "A million things can get in the way of your good night's sleep," says Shelby Harris, PsyD, director of the behavioral medicine program at the Montefiore Sleep-Wake Disorders Center in New York City. "Anything that causes stress can disrupt your sleep—even good things, like getting married or having a baby." On the short list of sleep-wrecking problems, Dr. Harris lists stress, too much on your schedule, a divorce, job or money troubles, menopause and its hot flashes, medical problems, and chronic pain, especially fibromyalgia and migraines.

According to a 2011 poll by the National Sleep Foundation, a nonprofit dedicated to sleep research, 43 percent of people say they "rarely or never" get a good night's sleep on weeknights. And 15 percent report getting fewer than 6 hours of sleep on weeknights—an amount that research shows can lead to obesity and chronic diseases.

Our understanding of sleep disorders is changing so rapidly that even the mental health industry is having a hard time keeping up with the developments. In fact, the upcoming *Diagnostic and Statistical Manual of Mental Diseases* (DSM)—the "bible" for mental health professionals—will list at least 10 new sleep disorder classifications and remove others from the manual.

Officially, sleep problems fall into two groups: dysomnias and parasomnias. The first group includes problems with getting enough sleep at the right time. But parasomnias relate to unusual—and unwanted—behavior that happens while you're sleeping. Here's the rundown:

Primary insomnia. Simply put, this means difficulty getting to sleep or staying asleep. This is the category that most people, and probably you, fall into. It becomes an official disorder when sleep loss is severe enough to disturb daytime functioning and well-being. The good news is that most of the sleep tips given in this chapter will help with all three of the following types (though you may have more than one):

- *Sleep-onset insomnia* is when you have trouble falling asleep.

- *Sleep-maintenance insomnia* is difficulty staying asleep.

- *Terminal insomnia* is when you wake too early and can't get back to sleep.

Beyond these three types of insomnia are several sleep disorders that are more complicated and require professional treatment. They include:

Primary hypersomnia. This is excessive daytime—or nighttime—sleepiness. People who sleep more than 10 hours at night and have a really hard time waking up in the morning or people who nod off excessively during the day are said to have this condition. Primary hypersomnia is a serious disorder that interferes with a person's ability to hold a job or otherwise function in daily life. Though behavioral therapies and sleep hygiene solutions generally aren't very helpful for this condition, scheduling naps at times recommended by your doctor and taking medication can effectively treat it.

Narcolepsy. If you suddenly fall into the sleep state in which dreams occur (called rapid eye movement sleep, or REM) while you're awake, you're likely to be diagnosed with this chronic sleep disorder. People with narcolepsy can fall asleep when they're driving, at work or school, and even in the middle of a meal or a conversation. Daytime sleepiness is one symptom; others include a sudden loss in muscle tone (cataplexy), vivid hallucinations, and moments of total paralysis. This scary and potentially dangerous condition (narcolepsy sufferers can injure themselves or others if it happens while they're driving or operating dangerous machinery) is caused by the brain's inability to regulate the body's sleep-wake cycles, possibly due to a genetic disturbance or other brain abnormality. Though narcolepsy isn't rare (it affects about 1 in 2,000 American adults), sleep professionals say that it's underrecognized and underdiagnosed. Your doctor will recommend scheduled naps and help you structure a sleeping schedule that works for you. For mild cases, that may be all you need to overcome narcolepsy, though more serious cases would probably require medication.

Breathing-related sleep disorder. If you have trouble breathing properly at night, you're not going to get a good night's sleep. Various conditions fall into this category, including sleep apnea, in which a person literally stops breathing for seconds at a time, causing the sleeper to wake repeatedly during the night, resulting in very poor sleep quality. People with sleep apnea often feel tired and sleepy during the day, and the condition has also been linked to obesity. It can be caused either by a physical obstruction of the upper airway or by a problem with the brain's respiration center. Treating sleep-related breathing problems starts with getting a comprehensive sleep evaluation. Talk to your health care provider about getting a referral to a sleep specialist. Sleep apnea is usually resolved with Continuous Positive Airway Pressure (CPAP) therapy. A CPAP machine, which is used while you sleep, forces oxygen into your airways at a high enough pressure to keep them open so you don't have breathing interruptions.

Circadian rhythm sleep disorder. Disruptions to your body clock can result in four sleep rhythm problems. (See Chapter 4 for more details.)

Nightmare disorder is a chronic problem marked by nightmares that wake you repeatedly during the night. Fifty percent of adults are troubled by sleep-disrupting nightmares. If you have dreams that trouble you regularly, the first thing to do is to faithfully follow the sleep hygiene tips starting on page 47. Don't nap during the day, and do some aerobic exercise 4 hours before bedtime. Avoid caffeine, alcohol, and cigarettes. Make sure to get to bed at the same time every night and to wake up at the same time each morning, and calm your mood by meditating or using progressive relaxation, which is described on page 50. If you're still having nightmares after following these tips for 2 to 3 weeks, see your doctor—he or she may prescribe anti-anxiety or tranquilizing medications.

Night (or sleep) terrors disorder is much more common in young children than in adults—but if your child suffers from this condition, your sleep will certainly be disrupted, too. (Once you've been awakened by the sound of your kid screaming bloody murder in the middle of the night, you're pretty much shot, sleepwise, for the rest of the night.) Up to 50 percent of children ages 3 to 5 will experience night terrors. Typical signs include screaming during the night and waking up in a panic, and it usually occurs about 90 minutes after they've fallen asleep. Your child may be confused, unresponsive, disoriented, or unable to tell you what happened, and may even wet the bed. The good news: Nearly all kids grow out of night terrors.

Restless leg syndrome (RLS) is an equal-opportunity sleep-buster: It wakes you whether you or your partner has it. RLS is common but is considered underdiagnosed, affecting somewhere between 5 and 10 percent of adults. Remember Kramer's "She's got the jimmy legs" line from an episode of *Seinfeld?* Funny as it was, it put a too light spin on a troubling problem—the tingling, prickly leg sensation causes sufferers to involuntarily move or even thrash their legs around at night to get relief, ruining their sleep and their partner's. RLS is associated with depression and even panic attacks. If you or your partner has RLS, see your doctor to rule out possible causes such as anemia or varicose veins. Then attack any bad habits that may be behind it. If you're a smoker, stop—that alone can slash symptoms, as can avoiding caffeine and alcohol. Daily daytime exercise will also help. If it persists, ask your doctor about prescribing medication.

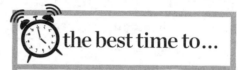 **the best time to...**

TAKE HEART MEDS

A 2010 study in Spain found that taking blood pressure medicine before bed rather than in the morning made it more effective in reducing blood pressure. Subjects who took at least one of their blood pressure meds at night suffered a third as many strokes, heart attacks, and other cardiovascular events as those who took their meds in the morning. Likewise, statins taken before bed will be most active during the night, giving cholesterol production a boost. Of course, check with your doctor before changing your medication schedule.

Lose Weight in the Dark

When we think about getting a good night's sleep, several key elements come to mind: silence; a cozy, comfortable bed; and, of course, darkness. But what you may not realize is how serious you have to be about enforcing a strict "lights out" policy in the bedroom.

Here's why: Melatonin (the sleep hormone) is produced in your pineal gland only when it's dark. This tiny, pinecone-shaped gland is only about as big as a grain of rice. But its importance to your sleep is enormous.

Located in the bottom front part of your brain, the pineal gland knows when it's dark because it picks up light signals transmitted from your retina (even when your eyes are closed, which is why light can trigger the wake-up process while you are still asleep). These signals activate the pineal gland to ramp up melatonin production and secretion, a job it does as long as the darkness lasts—the longer the darkness, the longer that melatonin is produced. The process shuts down when it gets light, so you start to wake up.

Though morning light is designed to shut off melatonin production, any light will slow or stop its flow. This means that if you wake up in the night and turn on the lights, the TV, or even the bathroom light for as long as it takes you to tinkle—poof! Your melatonin production levels plummet. You've shot yourself in the foot, sleepwise, because secretion of the hormone ceases. What's more, hormones such as cortisol that wake you up begin circulating through your system, hitting you with a double whammy of sleeplessness.

In fact, melatonin production is suppressed within minutes of exposure to bright light. And other research suggests that bright light, compared with dim light, activates your central nervous system. Indeed, exposure to artificial Light at Night (LAN) cancels out the sun's natural setting time in your internal clock and could harm your ability both to get to sleep and to stay asleep. In two British studies published in the *Abstract of Clinical Endocrinology and Metabolism,* participants were exposed to either room light or dim light during the 8 hours before bedtime. Compared with dim light, room light was associated with a later onset of melatonin production (which usually starts around 9:00 p.m.) in 99 percent of the subjects, and their melatonin production lasted about 90 minutes less. When they were exposed to room light during sleep hours, their melatonin production decreased by more than 50 percent.

Our constant exposure to high levels of light disrupts our internal clock and can damage the circadian regulation of cells, tissues, organs, and bodily systems. If exposure to light at night is knocking you off your sleep patterns and, therefore, your circadian rhythm, it's knocking you off your weight loss program too.

Could Night Light Be Making You Fat?

In 2010, a group of neuroscientists from the University of Ohio and the University of Haifa in Israel collaborated on a very interesting piece of research. The scientists subjected groups of mice to three different light environments. The first group was exposed to regular light/dark cycles—16 hours of bright light and 8 hours of darkness. The second group had 16 hours of bright light and 8 hours of dim light (equal to the light of five candles). And the third group was placed in a setting of continuous brightness (equal to 150 candles). All the mice had access to food and water and maintained their usual sleep patterns.

After 6 weeks, the mice exposed to more light were much heavier (they gained 50 percent more weight) than the mice in normal day/night environments— even though the groups ate and exercised the same. Researchers believe that the light exposure messed up the mice's biological clocks and their hormonal signals for feeding. (The mice exposed to light ate more than half their food at times when they should have been resting.) Other studies have hinted that *when* you take in your calories can also impact how much weight you gain.

(continued on page 44)

My Belly Melt

"This program busted me out of a weight loss standstill!"

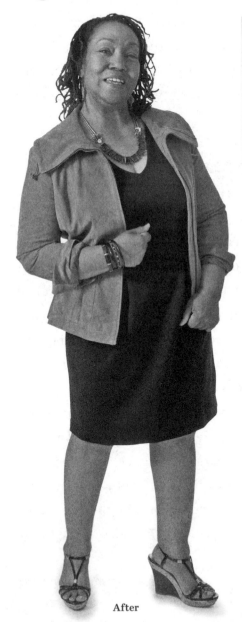

After

Mary Davis

AGE: 62

POUNDS LOST: 8.2 in 35 days

POUNDS LOST IN 3-DAY RESET: 3

ALLOVER INCHES LOST: 9

INCHES FROM WAIST LOST: 4

BODY FAT LOST: 2.3 percent

At the end of 5 weeks, a lighter, happier Mary beams. She's more than 8 pounds lighter, and reports record-setting confidence and energy (in fact, she rated her post-test energy and confidence as "11" on a scale of 1 to 10). When she started the BMD program, she was in that tough spot we all dread: at a weight loss plateau. "I had lost 30 pounds, but I was stuck. For 5 weeks, I hadn't lost a single pound."

The program got her back on track. The day after her orientation, she bought the eye shades and earplugs. The result? "When I left here the first night of the diet, it was the best night of sleep I'd had in ages. I bought

Success Story

the blinders and used earplugs. I was afraid I wouldn't hear sounds that I needed to hear, but it worked so well, it was all right."

As for food, Mary finally found the antidote for her cravings: When the sugar monster struck, she sipped a BMD Crave-Reducing Shake (find the recipe on page 231). The sweetness of the banana, plus the kale or collard juice she added, "made me okay," she says.

Exercise was doing the trick, too. "Karen Posten (profile on page 112) and I would walk together every morning," she says. Mary loved how their 6:00 a.m. walks jump-started her day. And to make the walk even more enjoyable, the two took a bird song class so that they could identify the calls on their walks. "We learned to recognize bird songs. There's a rabbit who waits for us every morning, and on the way home, a tree dropped a carpet of red berries on the ground."

As time went on, Mary found that she was stock-piling healthful food everywhere: "I had carrots at my desk, Gala apples and Asian pears in my car, and mini whole wheat pitas at my mother's house." She carries fresh ginger to chew throughout the day. "People laugh and say, 'Why do you have all this food? Aren't you on a diet?'

"I like the food plan—you don't feel hungry," Mary continues. "The portions are fine. And now it's like *boom!* I have the sense of how much to eat. When I went out to a restaurant and stuck to what I should eat, I took so much food home, it fed me for 3 days."

Toward the end of the 5 weeks, her 92-year-old mother fell. Luckily, no bones were broken, but Mary spent hours in the hospital while the doctors examined her mom. That's when she knew that the eating plan had become second nature: Even with all the stress, she wasn't tempted to eat emotionally.

"I can see my stomach coming down," Mary says—and she's not the only one who's noticed. "I'm single. At Bible study last week, a man came in and said, 'Oooh, Mary, you lost some weight.' I was trying to be cool, but inside I was saying, '*Yes!*'"

Before

Even a small amount of light at night adds to weight gain in mice, says neuroscientist Laura Fonken, a graduate student in Ohio State University's behavioral neuroscience program, who studies light's effects on eating habits. And it may have the same effect on people. "Turning on the light to read in the middle of the night can suppress melatonin," Fonken says. What's more, the brighter the light, the more that melatonin levels are suppressed.

This research could help connect the dots between our increasing exposure to artificial light at night and the growing epidemic of obesity in people. Think about it: Until the 20th century, people went to bed when it got dark and woke when it was light. They had no lamps, TVs, or iPads to keep them awake half the night. They got more sleep, and guess what else? They were thinner.

Let There Be Darkness

So you get the point: The more pitch-black your bedroom is, the better you'll be able to sleep. Which is why going dark in your bedroom is the first important step of the Belly Melt Diet. This simple step may be the easiest thing you can do to help you sleep better and lose more weight.

- First, go into your bedroom at night with the lights out and inspect it, taking a close look at any light sources. Seek out all sources of electronic light, and remove or cover them. If you have a lighted alarm clock, turn it away from the bed or cover it to block the light. Yes, even that light can disrupt your slumber (and who wants to be staring at it at 3:00 a.m., when you can't get to sleep?).

- If necessary, install room-darkening shades or curtains. This is especially helpful for people who wake up too early because of natural light entering the bedroom.

- Buy an eye mask to wear at night. Belly Melt panelist Mary Davis (see her full story on page 42) said that this alone made an amazing difference in the quality of her sleep.

Turn Off the iPad, the BlackBerry, and the Laptop . . .

Thanks to their portable size and Wi-Fi capabilities, electronic devices have crept into the bedroom. It's just so tempting to check your e-mail one last time or check the next day's weather from your bed. And we're all doing it: A 2011 Sleep in America poll by the National Sleep Foundation revealed that a stunning 95 percent of those polled say that they watch TV, play electronic games, or use computers, cell phones, e-readers or similar devices right before bed.

But here's why that's a bad idea in terms of getting a good night's sleep and staying slim (apart from the fact that reading a flaming e-mail from your boss at 11:00 p.m. will no doubt keep you up all night): "These devices cast a bluish light, which is even more disruptive to melatonin production than full-spectrum light," Charles Czeisler, MD, PhD, of Harvard Medical School and a Sleep in America 2011 task force member, said in the sleep report. That's right—the light from laptops and Smartphones is worse for your circadian rhythm than the light from a lamp. "This study reveals that light-emitting screens are in heavy use within the pivotal hour before we go to sleep," added Dr. Czeisler in the report. "Invasion of such alerting technologies into the bedroom may explain why so many people routinely get less sleep than they need." So take your last look at least an hour (preferably 2 hours) before bed, and then keep them out of your bedroom so you're not tempted to check.

Another reason to turn off your cell phone? Swedish researchers studied more than 4,100 young adults and found that those who reported frequent mobile phone use had a higher risk of being stressed and having sleeping problems. Frequent phone use also increased the risk of developing sleep disturbances (and you gotta hate those wrong-number calls at 2:00 in the morning).

- Move the TV and computer out of the bedroom. The light that these devices emit not only messes up your melatonin production but can keep you from going to sleep at an earlier hour. We mean, really, was watching Jay Leno worth your being exhausted—and possibly heavier— this morning?

- Close your bedroom door to keep any hallway or bathroom light from filtering in.

Dim All the Lights

Your bedroom is ready for a dark and comfortable night's sleep—now it's time to get your body ready. Not all of us are adversely affected by living in an environment that's artificially illuminated 24/7. But if you have trouble getting a good night's sleep, it's possible that your internal clock has been deleteriously impaired by artificial nighttime light. Here's a light-based strategy that will virtually guarantee you get the darkness you need.

- As you read earlier, melatonin production starts around 9:00 p.m., and you can help it along by starting your lights-out bedtime ritual around that time. About an hour or so before bed (2 hours, if you find that you have a really hard time getting to sleep), shut off the TV and use dimmer lights or lower the strength of the lights you have around the house. Read or do some other relaxing activity using a low-wattage side lamp.

- So that you don't kill yourself getting up to go to the bathroom in the middle of the night, invest in low-wattage amber night lights, and use them in the bedroom, bathroom, and hallways from 9:00 p.m. until the morning. Why amber? Because the "blue" component of light rays shuts off melatonin production. If you like to read in bed, you can also find amber bulbs for your bedside lamp (but remember, no Kindles!).

- If you just can't live without *CSI* and must watch TV after 9:00, don a pair of amber eye shades. These inexpensive glasses (you can find styles that fit over regular eyeglasses) block blue light. You may even want to get a blue-light-blocking filter to fit over your computer screen; you can find this at www.lowbluelights.com.

Clean Up Your Sleep Act

Now that we have the number one factor in getting a good night's sleep taken care of, let's look at the other ways to get restful shut-eye. "Sleep hygiene" has nothing to do with washing your face and brushing your teeth before you hit the sack. But it has everything to do with helping you to fall asleep and stay asleep once you get there. Sleep hygiene is an umbrella term that covers the basic habits you need to follow to get a really good night's sleep—every night. Take this boot camp approach—not all of these strategies will be easy to follow, but they'll virtually guarantee sleep success if you're persistent.

Set the same bedtime and wake time. And be a fanatic about it—even on weekends. Sleep experts say that you "entrain" your body to sleep cues, which means you'll get used to sleeping and waking at the same time every

Enjoy the Sound of Silence

Noise pollution—especially from road, air, and rail traffic—can seriously disrupt your sleep, says Mathias Basner, MD, assistant professor of sleep and chronobiology in psychiatry at the University of Pennsylvania School of Medicine in Philadelphia. That noise disturbs sleep seems like a no-brainer—but the reasons may surprise you. Because noise is potentially associated with danger, it subtly activates your central nervous system via heart rate increases and changes in brain activity. Not so subtly, loud noises can rouse you from a deep sleep and make you fully awake. "Loud noises can fragment your sleep and make it less recuperative than undisturbed sleep," Dr. Basner says.

What's more, low noise may even disrupt the circadian cycles in some sensitive people. "Some research shows that noise levels above 55 decibels are potent enough to disturb sleep," he adds. That's roughly the same noise level as an air-conditioning unit 100 feet away or restaurant conversation—not much at all. If you're extremely sensitive to sound, consider installing sound-insulating windows, and keep them closed at night. Invest in earplugs, which can range from a few dollars in a drugstore to a nice chunk of change if you have them custom-made.

day if your sleep/wake times are the same every day. If you're a parent, you've seen this principle in action: When you've been persistent about putting your baby on a schedule, she usually sticks pretty close to it once you've enforced it for a couple of weeks.

Only power naps allowed. Don't let yourself fall into the trap of taking long, luxurious naps on the weekend unless you've got the flu or other illness. Otherwise, sleeping at night will become mission impossible. In "Take a Power Nap," you'll learn how this kind of nap will enhance your sleep at night instead of ruining it.

Rip up your worries. Rather than engaging your "hamster brain" as you fall asleep—when you lie in bed allowing your worries to wreak havoc in your brain—take control of your concerns. Spend a few minutes before bed writing your worries on a pad, as you tell yourself that you'll work on each problem the next day. You might find it helpful to put the pad or list in a drawer, and then close the drawer firmly.

Leave the bed. If you haven't fallen asleep within 15 to 20 minutes, haul yourself out of bed and go to another room (not—repeat, not—the kitchen). This will help because when you associate your bed only with sleeping and sex, you'll cue yourself, in a Pavlov's dog kind of way, to become sleepy (or amorous?) once you hit the mattress. With the lights dimmed as low as possible, read quietly, knit or crochet, or work easy puzzles until you feel sleepy again. Do not turn on the TV or use a computer or any handheld devices!

Read your body's thermostat. While there's no one-size-fits-all optimal temperature to sleep by, most people find that they sleep better in a slightly cool room. That's because your body temperature's set point (the temperature your internal thermostat maintains) goes down a little at night. But if your bedroom is too cold or too hot—for you—your sleep may be disturbed because your body will work to maintain its set point. Your best room temp might be anywhere from 60 to 72 degrees.

Take a Power Nap

If you've had a rough night of sleeplessness, a 15- to 20-minute midafternoon snooze-a-thon can ramp up alertness without impairing your natural rhythm or affecting your ability to sleep that night. The key? Make it a true catnap, lasting no more than 20 minutes.

- **Time it right.** Naps between 1:00 p.m. and 3:00 p.m. won't interfere with nighttime sleep, but later naps may.
- **Set your alarm for 20 minutes.** Going over that time will send you into a deeper sleep cycle, making it hard to wake up and even harder to get to sleep that night.
- **Sleep in a dark room or wear an eye mask**—you'll fall asleep faster when the lights are out.
- **Use a toasty blankie to keep you warm and cozy** (remember, your body temperature drops as you snooze).

Check your bedding. Intuitively, it makes perfect sense to think that your uncomfortable old mattress is ruining your restful zzz's. And according to studies, your intuition is right on the money: At least one researcher concludes in three different studies that new bedding can improve sleep and ease back pain, and that sleeping through the night may depend on getting a new mattress. Full disclosure: The researcher's studies were funded by the mattress industry. Still, if your mattress is aging, replacing it along with your scratchy sheets and lumpy pillows may improve the quality of your sleep— and replacing a sagging mattress with a new, firmer one could help alleviate minor back pain that interrupts sleep.

Kick out any hairy guests. By this we mean Fido and Fluffy. If you share a bedroom with your pets and they bother you at night, send them packing. Yes, we know this is easier said than done. Enlist the aid of a trainer if necessary, and be patient for a couple of weeks as both of you learn to adjust.

When the Other Person in the Bed
Is Keeping You Up

If your partner is a chronic snorer, you may have more than a noise problem on your hands, says David O. Volpi, MD, founder of the Manhattan Snoring and Sleep Center in New York City. "Snoring can be a sign of sleep apnea, which has potentially serious health consequences, including high blood pressure, heart problems, and daytime sleepiness. In fact, people with sleep apnea often awake feeling so sleepy that they pose a risk to themselves and others when they drive." The same goes for the sleep-deprived partner of a snorer, says Dr. Volpi. Unsurprisingly, being overweight can contribute to sleep apnea. In a recent study from researchers of Karolinska Institute in Sweden, overweight and obese men who lost weight on a calorie-restricted diet over 9 weeks saw major improvements in their sleep apnea and were able to maintain those changes up to a year later. If you or your partner have obesity-driven sleep apnea, the Belly Melt Diet will not only help you slim down, but may also help you reclaim a good night's sleep—every night.

Since other health issues can contribute to snoring, such as having a deviated septum, he recommends seeing a sleep specialist to have the snoring evaluated.

And if your doctor-phobic partner resists your suggestion that he or she be evaluated? You have to take matters into your own hands, says Dr. Volpi. The most effective move you can make is into the guest bedroom. "When a wife tells her husband she won't sleep with him until he gets his snoring checked out, it's a pretty powerful impetus."

Relax First, Then Sleep

According to sleep specialists at the Sleep Disorders Center at the University of Maryland Medical Center, relaxation techniques can help resolve sleep problems when practiced faithfully. This technique, called progressive relaxation, is an especially effective way to ease yourself into blessed oblivion.

Make it part of your sleep ritual, and before you know it, it will become ingrained in your own cycle.

- Lie on your back and close your eyes. Direct your consciousness to your feet. Mentally sense them, and tense them slightly. Then, starting with each toe, relax all the little muscles, and sink into bed. Progress to your ankles, feeling their joints and relaxing them.

- Move up your shins to your knees, mentally relaxing your muscles and even your skin, slowly and methodically. Feel them sink into the bed. Next, relax your hips and thighs, and feel as they become heavy and sink into the bed.

The Down Under Way to Stop Snoring

Whether it's you or your partner who wakes the dead with nighttime snoring, try this toning exercise, which is based on playing the didgeridoo, the Australian musical instrument (that weird noise you hear in those Outback commercials). In what has to be one of the oddest studies we've come across, Swiss researchers assigned 25 snorers with sleep apnea to one of two groups: One group took didgeridoo lessons, while the other was put on a waiting list for lessons. Not only did the didgeridoo players sleep better and snore less, but their partners reported sleeping better, too. The researchers chalked the improvements up to the fact that playing the didgeridoo (hopefully not at night—these instruments sound about as relaxing as, say, bagpipes) can tone and train your upper airways, and thus lessen snoring. No didgeridoo handy? This easy exercise will help you tone and strengthen your antisnoring muscles in pretty much the same way.

- Tap your tongue against the roof of your mouth over and over.

- While you're tapping, chant nonsense sounds.

- Pull your tongue toward the back of your mouth and swallow while doing the first 2 steps.

Train for about 5 minutes a day, and be patient. In a couple of months, you're likely to find yourself a quieter sleeper—and a great didgeridoo player.

- Direct your consciousness up through your belly and into your chest. Breathe deeply into your abdomen, feeling it rise as you do. Deepen and slow your breathing, and feel your belly and chest sink into the bed.

- Feel your buttocks and the muscles in your lower back. Consciously relax all those tense muscles, letting them sink into the bed. As you move up your back, relax every muscle all the way up to your neck, then relax your back and let it sink into the bed.

- Now, focus attention on your neck and shoulders. Note any tense spots and consciously relax them. Continue to breathe deeply, and let your neck and shoulders relax and sink into the bed.

- Feel your head. Relax all the muscles in your scalp, your forehead, your face. Let your skull sink into the bed. Relax your mouth and jaw. Unclench your jaw muscles if they feel tight. Feel your mouth and jaw relax and sink into the bed.

- Now, scan your entire body, looking for any last vestiges of tension. Relax those spots, breathe deeply, and drift off to sleep.

Go to Sleep, Naturally

So you've turned your bedroom into a dark, cool, quiet cave. You've stepped away from the electronic gizmos—and by that we mean TV too—for at least an hour before bed. Despite your best efforts, though, when you hit the pillow, you still can't sleep. Or you fall asleep just fine, but wake wide-eyed hours later.

Clearly, you need extra help. While medication can help, most experts agree that it's only for short-term use, as it can screw up your internal cycle and even be addictive. Instead, try these natural sleep aids that should soothe you into slumber land.

Chamomile tea. This delicate apple-scented tea is gentle enough to drink every night before bed and, in fact, is great as part of a relaxing presleep ritual. Its use for easing anxiety and soothing a nervous stomach goes back centuries, and chamomile may be all you need to bring on restful sleep. Use two tea bags per cup of boiled water, cover the cup, and let steep for 15 minutes before sipping.

Melatonin. The hormone supplement can help you sleep, especially if your sleeplessness is connected to circadian rhythm issues like jet lag or seasonal affective disorder (SAD), or if you work a late shift. It can also help with age-related insomnia. Find melatonin in health food and drugstores. For common insomnia, take up to 1 milligram an hour before bedtime. Larger doses aren't any more effective, and slow-release melatonin isn't as effective as the fast-release melatonin tablets.

Passionflower. If worries and stress keep you awake at night, consider giving this herbal sedative a try. In at least one study, passionflower was as effective as the prescription tranquilizer Serax (oxazepam) after a month of treatment, plus it didn't cause the on-the-job performance problems that the drug did. Two other clinical trials, including a 2008 study, found that passionflower can significantly lower anxiety. You can find it in health food stores in capsules, and as liquid tinctures. Take a teaspoon of passionflower tincture up to four times daily, including an hour before bedtime.

Valerian. People the world over have relied on slightly smelly valerian to ease them safely to sleep for centuries. In a 2011 Mayo Clinic study, researchers gave cancer survivors with insomnia either valerian or a placebo for 8 weeks. The participants said they had less trouble with sleeping and didn't feel drowsy the next morning after they took valerian. Take 400 to 800 milligrams (capsules) or 1 teaspoon of valerian tincture an hour before bedtime. Good brands to try include Herbalist & Alchemist and HerbPharm for tinctures, and GNC or Vitamin Shoppe for capsules.

Eat to Sleep

If you're even the tiniest bit sleep-conscious, you probably know better than to drink coffee in the evening or tuck into chili as a late-night snack. Coffee can keep you up way past the 11:00 o'clock news, and chili creates that hot lava monster within called heartburn, another sleep disrupter. But you may be surprised by the other foods that can keep you tossing and turning all night as if you had a double shot of espresso at midnight.

Alcohol. When you booze, you don't snooze. Alcohol tampers with your body clock in many different ways, by sending you conflicting messages. First, it lowers your body temperature, a natural clue that tells you to nod off; that and its sedative effect are what make you ready to doze after a few drinks. But then, a few hours later, you get a rebound rise in temperature, something that doesn't usually happen until 4:00 to 5:00 a.m. And your sleep cycles—both restorative REM (rapid eye movement) sleep and non-REM sleep—are disturbed. Those drinks that put you to sleep are now waking you up several times during the night like a rude poke, particularly during the restorative REM periods, while increasing the amount of light, or superficial, sleep you have. The next morning you can feel like you've pulled an all-nighter.

Unfortunately for women, this is more often the case for them than for their male counterparts: A study published in the *Abstract of Alcoholism* found that women reported greater sleeplessness, slept fewer hours, woke more frequently, and had more disrupted sleep than men had after drinking alcohol.

And more than just ruining your sleep, it affects your weight loss efforts: Alcohol triggers your body to produce galanin, a hormone that makes you want more alcohol and—oh, while you're at it—something fatty to eat. Alcohol also inhibits the secretion of leptin, the hormone that keeps your cravings in check, which may explain why a couple of glasses of wine make the fried mozzarella sticks appetizer look so darn good.

High-fat diet. When researchers looked at the diets of nearly 500 women in the Women's Health Initiative—the largest study of its kind looking at women's health—they found that the sleepiest women also had the most fat in their diets. Fat even scored higher than caffeine as a sleep disrupter!

A Brazilian study found that too many superfat meals will have you waking up many times throughout the night, and when you do catch a few zzz's, they're unlikely to be REM sleep, the refreshing sleep phase when you dream. Even more disturbing, people in the study who ate a lot of fat were more likely to have breathing problems at night—the kind that characterize obstructive sleep apnea, a condition in which the sleeper stops breathing up to hundreds of times a night, waking him or her.

A high-fat diet can also reset your clock in ways that affect more than your sleep. In an Israeli study, researchers fed mice either a low-fat or a high-fat diet, followed by a fasting day, and measured levels all along what's known as the adiponectin signaling pathway. Adiponectin is a hormone secreted by fat cells that regulates how your body metabolizes glucose and fats and determines how your cells respond to insulin, the hormone that helps them use the energy from your diet as fuel.

The researchers found that after gorging on fat, the mice's little biological clocks went into a phase delay—the timing of their metabolic processes was off, as was the daily rhythm of their clock genes, which regulate the production of proteins and hormones and govern the sleep/wake cycle, and, like a stellar administrative assistant, the body's entire schedule. That fat gorge also inhibited the production of adiponectin—a dieter's best friend. Researchers at the University of Pennsylvania found that adiponectin can raise your metabolic rate—that is, the rate at which you burn calories. In their study with mice, those given an injection of the hormone ate the same number of calories as their cohorts that didn't get the injection, but they lost weight—by burning it off. Many overweight and obese people have low levels of adiponectin.

The Diet That Helps You Doze

Though we know more about the foods that keep us up, there are some that help us sleep, too. If this makes you think of a glass of warm milk, you're in for a surprise. Even though that's the best-known sleep aid of all time, there's really no evidence that it acts as anything more than a placebo to help you nod off.

Yes, milk has a minute amount of melatonin, the sleep hormone, but by itself it's probably not enough to conk you out. And, yes, milk contains tryptophan, the amino acid your brain uses to make serotonin, the raw material for melatonin. The problem is, high-protein foods like milk contain other substances that can block tryptophan from going on its appointed rounds to your brain—notably tyrosine, another amino acid found in protein that will actually rev you up.

In fact, if you want to make tryptophan, you need carbs. A 2003 study by researchers at the Massachusetts Institute of Technology found that pairing carbohydrates with milk triggered the production of insulin, which makes it easier for the tryptophan to enter your brain. So if you're going to try warm milk, make it low-fat or nonfat (fat impairs sleep), and pair it with a cookie or another carb.

That's right, we just gave you permission to eat a cookie—as your nighttime snack. If you're going to eat sweets, bedtime's the time. In a study published in the *American Journal of Clinical Nutrition,* researchers from the School of Exercise and Sport Science at the University of Sydney found that eating a food high on the glycemic index (GI)—a measure of how much a food you consume will raise your blood sugar—can help you get to sleep faster. In the study, people who ate a high-GI snack (in this case, a bowl of Jasmine rice with steamed vegetables and tomato puree) had a spike in blood sugar and insulin, and fell asleep almost 50 percent earlier than they did after eating a low-GI meal.

A healthier nighttime snack would be a bowl of oatmeal, cereal with low-fat milk, low- or nonfat yogurt, or a slice of whole wheat toast spread with natural peanut butter and sliced banana (which contains tryptophan and the muscle-relaxing minerals potassium and magnesium).

Cherry-Pick Your Snacks

Around bedtime, munch on a few tart Montmorency cherries. These cherries are one of a number of plant-based sources of melatonin, the sleep hormone. (Bananas and corn have it, too.) While there's no evidence that they'll help you nod off, studies have found that foods like these can raise melatonin levels in the body. Not only does melatonin help you sleep, but it's a powerful antioxidant that can protect your cells from free radical damage, the kind that leads to cancer, Alzheimer's, and other diseases. That should help you sleep easy. Not a fan of cherries? Drink the juice. In a small study conducted by researchers at the University of Pennsylvania, the University of Rochester, and the Canandaigua VA Medical Center, people who drank 8 ounces of the tart cherry (also known as sour cherry) juice in the morning and another 8 ounces in the evening for 2 weeks reported better sleeping habits.

If reading about all these foods is putting you to sleep, never fear. The Belly Melt Diet Reset starting on page 115 takes all this into account, providing you with the ideal mix of food that not only will help you lose weight without cravings but will also maximize your energy during the day and help you wind down naturally to sleep well at night.

Help! I've Fallen Asleep and I Can't Wake Up!

So now you have the going-to-sleep part under control, but then the morning arrives, and the idea of waking up seems like a nightmare. Well, just as you shut out the light to get to sleep, you need to expose yourself to light to wake up. But, of course, we've just told you to make your room as dark as a tomb. To wake up the slow and steady way, treat yourself to a dawn simulator, bedside lights that can be set like an alarm clock. Start with a low-dose light, slowly—and we mean s-l-o-w-l-y—the light gets brighter as you get closer to your desired wake-up time. The light travels through your eyelids and tells

MEDITATION BEATS MEDICATION

Mindfulness-based stress reduction (MBSR) is an über-relaxing practice, developed about 20 years ago by Jon Kabat-Zinn, PhD, professor emeritus of medicine and the founding director of the Center for Mindfulness at the University of Massachusetts Medical School. The 8-week program is offered in many hospitals and YMCA/YWCAs. Unlike other forms of meditation, in which you focus your attention on your breath or on a mantra (a word or phrase that you chant silently), MBSR teaches you to sit quietly, focus only on the present moment, and note your thoughts without judging them.

Recently, researchers at Rush University Medical Center in Chicago studied a mindfulness-based approach to insomnia. Of the 30 people in their study, 15 experienced a 50 percent or better reduction in wake time, and at the end of the treatment, all but two were sleeping normally. After a year, 61 percent of the participants were still insomnia free. And in a 2011 study, University of Minnesota researchers assigned 30 people with chronic insomnia to one of two groups: One group underwent MBSR training for 8 weeks, and the other took the sleeping pill Lunesta (eszopiclone) every night for 8 weeks. At the end of the study, people in the MBSR group fell asleep faster than those in the medication group, and also chalked up major improvements in their overall sleep time.

And in news that astounded even the researchers themselves, a team from Massachusetts General Hospital reported their 2011 discovery that practicing MBSR for just 8 weeks actually changes the structure of the brain in a way that enhances well-being and quality of life.

your body to shut down melatonin production and ramp up your wake-up hormones, but it does it in a nice and calm manner. Find them at www.amazon.com for under $100.

Not up for that? You can do it the old-fashioned—and a bit more brutal—way. As you drag yourself out of bed, schlep over to the windows and pull up those light-blocking shades. You'll get a full—and a vampire painful—dose of daylight to get your wakey-wakey hormones moving.

When You Really Just Can't Get to Sleep

If you still have trouble getting to sleep after you've spent at least a week or so following our sleep suggestions, you need to step up your game. But rather than resorting to sleeping pills, work on changing your behavior, along with adopting relaxation techniques. The following methods, administered by licensed practitioners, have been proven to work:

Cognitive Behavior Therapy (CBT). In at least two clinical trials, this short-term (8 to 12 weekly sessions) talk-therapy approach has been proven to be more effective than sleeping pills at treating insomnia. A CBT therapist will coach you on how to sleep better by using approaches like the following, depending on your needs:

CAN NEEDLES PROMOTE ZZZ'S?

In a study by researchers from the University of Toronto and other Canadian institutions, published in the *Journal of Neuropsychiatry Clinical Neurosciences*, they found that acupuncture increases nighttime melatonin levels and reduces insomnia and anxiety. And in an extensive review of acupuncture studies, researchers at the University of Pittsburgh concluded that acupuncture may be an effective insomnia treatment.

Acupuncture is practically a mainstream medical practice these days, and thousands of clinical studies have shown it to be a useful treatment for pain and various other ailments. You can find MDs as well as licensed acupuncturists virtually anywhere—and the treatment is even covered by some insurance policies. Though there's still uncertainty about exactly how acupuncture works, researchers know that needling seems to ease anxiety by increasing levels of endorphins, those make-you-feel-good-all-over brain chemicals.

Psychotherapy and thought control. The therapist helps you examine the thoughts and worries that keep you awake at night. He or she will also help you explore false or scary beliefs you may have about sleep; once you do, you'll be better able to eliminate them.

Sleep restriction. If you wake up and stay awake in bed night after night, it can become a habit that's hard to break. The therapist may work with you to limit the amount of time you spend in bed so that you become sleepier and more likely to stay asleep when you do hit the sack.

Passive awakeness. Your therapist may coach you to avoid falling asleep, especially if worrying that you can't sleep is what's keeping you awake. If you let that worry drift away, as the CBT theory goes, you'll have a better chance of drifting off naturally.

Stimulus control therapy. This approach trains you, in a Pavlovian kind of way, to associate your bed with just two things: sleep and sex. The therapist may advise you to get out of bed after 15 minutes or so of sleeplessness and to return only when you're good and sleepy.

Breathe in the Lavender

Dorothy fell asleep strolling through fields filled with poppies in *The Wizard of Oz*—but lavender is the bloom that will really get your snooze on. At once bracing and delicate, lavender's nearly hypnotic fragrance comes from a complex marriage of plant chemicals with gentle sedative properties. Known for centuries for its powers to heal wounds and calm nerves, it's also a proven insomnia-easer in clinical studies. Keep a little bottle of the oil on your nightstand (find pure essential lavender oil, preferably organic, at a natural food store), and before you go to bed, sprinkle some on your pillowcase—and enjoy the *aahhhh* as you drift off. Resprinkle as needed during the night. (And don't worry—it won't stain your bed linens.)

Relaxation training. Your therapist will most likely cover the basics of several different relaxation techniques, including meditation and muscle relaxation. Some therapists may even use hypnosis training, which you can tap into when it's time to go to bed.

Biofeedback. With this approach, a therapist will set you up with a special device to take home, to measure your patterns of heart rate and muscle tension that can affect your sleep so that you can learn to help control them.

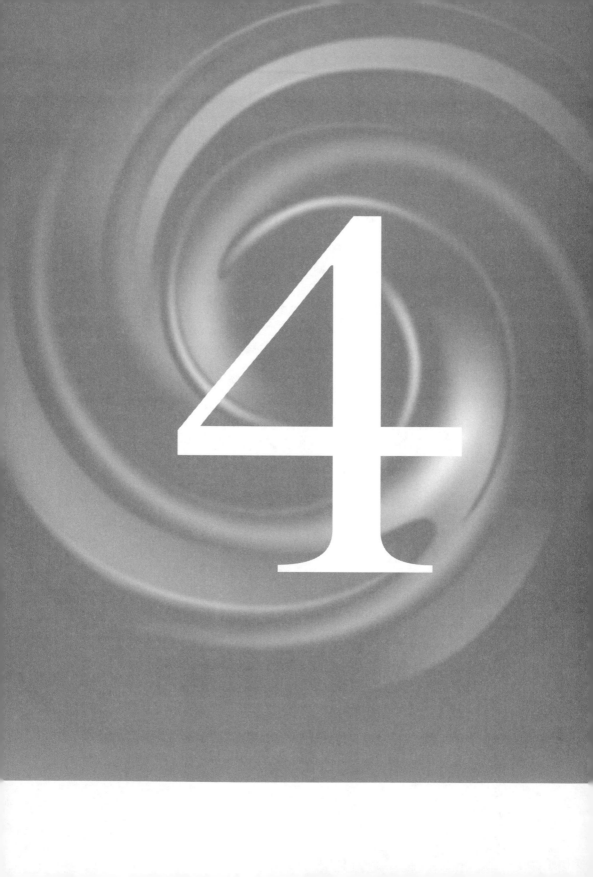

When Nighttime's a Nightmare

If you've faithfully adopted the sleep hygiene strategies outlined in Chapter 3 but still can't get your 40 winks, it's more likely that you have a circadian rhythm disorder rather than common insomnia, says sleep and circadian rhythm expert Bjørn Bjorvatn, MD, PhD, professor of general practice at Haukeland University Hospital in Bergan, Norway. Truth is, he says, most garden-variety insomnias tend to yield once you've battened down the hatches and put

A big part of the answer for treating out-of-whack circadian rhythm sleep problems is light therapy. Though there are several theories about exactly how light therapy works, there's not much doubt about its effectiveness, says Michael R. Privitera, MD, associate professor of psychiatry at the University of Rochester in New York. "Basically, light therapy replaces the light that's absent at certain times of the year," he says. "In the Northern Hemisphere, that time begins around October and ends in March." In his 2010 study published in the *Journal of Psychiatric Practice* on light therapy for symptoms of seasonal affective disorder—a.k.a. SAD, which can cause sleep problems—Dr. Privitera concluded that light therapy is a useful

SAD therapy. In fact, "some people have a milder version of SAD, where there are changes in sleep problems and increased appetite—without depression," he says. People with sleep and appetite problems who do not have depression also respond to light therapy, he says.

Light therapy may work by pushing your circadian rhythms forward, which in effect fools your body into falling into sleep at a more normal bedtime and sleeping more soundly, says Martha Howard, MD, the medical director of Wellness Associates in Chicago.

As therapies go, this one is as easy as pie (and no calories!). All you do is sit in front of a special light box for anywhere from 30 minutes to 2 hours a day—you may have to experiment a little with the

yourself on a better sleep schedule. But circadian rhythm sleep problems may resist even your best attempts to clean up your subpar bedtime habits.

And then there are those *other* cycles that some of us have to live with—menstrual and then menopause—that also have a field day with our sleep. Here we tackle issues and problems that go beyond basic insomnia.

Sleep Disorders and You

According to Dr. Bjorvatn and other sleep experts, circadian rhythm sleep disorders, which occur because of a glitch between the sleep cycles your body times, since there's no one-size-fits-all exposure time for everyone. Some people get relief from morning exposure, while others do best when they use it in the late afternoon or early evening, says Dr. Howard.

Light devices used to treat SAD (and other circadian rhythm imbalances that cause depression and sleep problems) have evolved and improved over the past 25 years. Now, new thinking about light boxes is trending away from the very large, full-spectrum devices that took up half your table. Newer light boxes are about the size of a smartphone, and are equally as effective at treating circadian-related sleep problems, says Dr. Howard. And since they are portable, you can use them anywhere, anytime.

Researchers at the University Center for Psychiatry in the Netherlands pitted one of these newer, smaller devices against the larger, standard model. Subjects suffering from major seasonal depression were treated for 22 days, and were assigned to either 30 minutes of therapy a day, 5 days a week, with the standard 10,000 lux model or with a smaller 750 lux model. After just 1 day of treatment, depression scores had decreased 76.4 percent in the group that used the 750 lux model and 65.2 percent in the group that used the 10,000 lux model. The model similar to the one used in the study is Philips GoLITE BLU, available at www.amazon.com for about $155. At just 7 inches square, it's small enough to sit next to your computer.

clock naturally imposes on you and the ones your daily life demands, require a special approach that includes specially timed bright-light treatment and, in some cases, specially timed doses of melatonin, the sleep hormone. Circadian rhythm disorders fall into six categories. Here's what you need to know about ID'ing and treating two key problems:

Delayed Sleep Phase Disorder (DSPD)

Nearly 1 out of 10 people who think they have insomnia actually have the circadian rhythm problem known as delayed sleep phase disorder, or DSPD. You could have DSPD if, despite your attempts to improve your sleep hygiene, you're still awake at night for hours and you need explosives to blast you awake in the morning. More ways to tell: If you had your druthers, you'd get to bed somewhere between 2:00 a.m. and 6:00 a.m., and wouldn't rise till noon—if then. This schedule suits you to a T—you get plenty of sleep and are refreshed when you finally wake up. The trouble is, of course, that this laid-back life plan doesn't cut it if your life includes a family or a job. So rather than getting to sleep late so you log a full night's shut-eye, you're hauling your butt out of bed when the alarm rings. You need buckets of coffee or even Red Bull to get your engine started. Once at work, you're groggy—maybe even grumpy—till 11:00 or so. Then the fog lifts, your energy ramps up, and your day begins.

Sleep experts suspect that these four factors—either singly or a combination of two or more—are responsible for DSPD:

It's your genes. You may have a genetic mutation that predisposes you to the disorder.

It's your rhythm. Your circadian rhythm cycle may simply be longer than normal.

It's your behavior. By keeping irregular hours, you could actually be training yourself to maintain an imperfect sleep schedule. It's very likely that these habits began in your teen or college years, and you just haven't outgrown your night owl ways.

It's the light. Some people are especially sensitive to the effects of light at night, which suppresses melatonin, the you-are-getting-sleepy hormone. The light—from room light, outdoor light seeping in through a window, a TV or computer screen—keeps you awake later. As a double whammy, by being a later riser, you miss being exposed to bright morning light, which triggers the wakey-wakey hormone, cortisol.

What to Do

Try as you might, you just can't fall asleep before the wee hours. To cope, you may look to sleeping pills to do the trick, but that's the wrong approach, say the sleep experts, since taking pills doesn't address the underlying issue: regulating your cycle. Instead, hit the override button.

First: Log (or blog) it. Use a sleep journal or blog to record your sleep activity for at least a week. That way, you can easily see if you have a consistent pattern of late-to-bed nights and late-to-rise mornings (or feeling exhausted when you do rise early). If that turns out to be your pattern, you need a combined approach of sleep hygiene tactics (see Chapter 3), timed bright-light therapy, and a nighttime dose of melatonin to reset your internal clock and find a pattern that works better for you.

Note: If you don't have to rise early for a job, kids, or other responsibilities (lucky person that you are) and you're getting 7 to 9 hours of shut-eye when you do sleep, then you don't have to retrain yourself to the rest of the world's sleep-wake cycles. Just don't let anyone call you a slacker!

The therapy. Take 5 milligrams of melatonin (available at health food stores and drugstores without a prescription) every night at 10:00 for 6 weeks. This is the timing and the dosage shown in at least one study to be successful, according to Northwestern University researchers in their 2010 review, "Therapeutics for Circadian Rhythm Sleep Disorders," published in *Sleep Medicine Clinics.* Even a year after using this 6-week melatonin treatment, 97 percent of people said their sleep habits had improved.

Try a dawn simulator. These bedside lamps on special timers help mend broken sleep cycles by recreating a gradual dawn. They slowly increase the light while you're sleeping and become fully bright as you're scheduled to wake up, says Michael R. Privitera, MD, associate professor of psychiatry at the University of Rochester in New York. See page 57 for more details.

Advanced Sleep Phase Disorder (ASPD)

This disorder, more common among older adults, means you fall asleep before TV's prime time begins and wake up way before the early-morning news shows come on. Even if you force yourself to stay awake long enough to have a normal family and social life, you'll still wake before dawn, usually before 5:00 a.m. Needless to say, as a result, you're exhausted and sleepy during the day. ASPD isn't a problem if your lifestyle can accommodate these unusual hours—but most people's lifestyles don't, so you need to take action before you fall asleep at your desk once too often. As with DSPD, experts aren't exactly sure what causes ASPD, though they suspect these factors may be involved:

It's your inheritance. Along with your height, hair color, and aptitude for algebra, you may have inherited this sleep pattern, which puts you out of sync with most of the rest of the world. It's due to a mutation in one of your clock genes, called hPER2, that's responsible for maintaining your circadian rhythm—and the mutation can be passed from generation to generation.

It's your body temperature. Your body temperature may cool too early and your melatonin levels may rise too early in the evening, which makes you sleepy long before a normal 10 p.m.-to-midnight bedtime.

It's your rhythm. This sleep-early/wake-early cycle may be due to your shorter than 24-hour circadian rhythm cycle.

What to Do

Just like with other circadian rhythm sleep-phase issues, the first step is to see if your sleep pattern is persistent for an extended period of time. Here's what you need to do:

First: Log (or blog) it. Use a sleep journal or blog to record your sleep activity for at least a week. (You can use the Belly Melt Diet journal pages found in the Appendix.) That way, you can clearly see if you have a consistent pattern of early-to-bed evenings combined with early-to-rise mornings. If you discover that your pattern mirrors that of ASPD—meaning that you tend to fall asleep around 8:00 at night and wake at 4:00 in the morning, give or take an hour on either side—you need a specially timed bright light. Using melatonin for treating ASPD is controversial, since the appropriate timing to make you sleep later dictates taking an early-morning dose. If you

WHEN YOU'RE REALLY LAGGING

Whether you're a seasoned traveler or an occasional tourist, jet lag can turn any trip or homecoming into a bit of a bummer. In a nutshell, the grogginess, sleepiness, and insomnia that greet you once you land several time zones away occur because your internal clock is out of sync with the actual clock at your destination. The more time zones you cross, the more disorienting your jet lag is likely to be. (It's easier to get in sync when you're traveling westbound than to points east.) Here's how to make every minute count:

DIM THE A.M. LIGHTS. Bright light, appropriately timed, can ease you into local time. For example, if you're flying from the East Coast of the United States to Paris, you're likely to arrive in the City of Light in the early morning. Don your darkest shades, hop a cab, and check in at your hotel, then rest in your darkened room for an hour or two. After your nap, lace up your most comfy walking shoes, and head outside to soak up all the bright late-morning and early-afternoon light you can get. Then proceed with a normal day- and nighttime schedule. (Travel hint: Before you go, ask your hotel for an early check-in.)

POP SOME MELATONIN. Once you arrive at your destination, the experts suggest taking 2 to 5 milligrams of melatonin before bedtime; you can take it for up to 4 days. In one study, people who took 5 milligrams of melatonin at 6:00 p.m. for 3 days before takeoff, followed by 4 days at bedtime (when traveling eastbound), rated their jet lag symptoms as less severe than did people in a control group, according to a 2010 Northwestern University review, "Therapeutics for Circadian Rhythm Sleep Disorders."

TRY PYCNOGENOL. This extract from a pine tree that grows only in the South of France decreased the severity and duration of jet lag symptoms in a 2008 study by researchers at the University of Chieti in Italy. Sixty-eight people took a 50-milligram pill or a placebo three times a day for 7 days, starting 2 days before takeoff. People in the Pycnogenol group reported that symptoms of jet lag lasted an average of 18.2 hours after their flight, compared with an average of 39.3 hours for those in the placebo group. You can find Pycnogenol at health food stores or online.

took melatonin, say, at 4:00 a.m., that might work if you're able to sleep until a normal wake-up time of between 7:00 and 8:00 a.m. But as some experts note, that could make you too sleepy to safely drive to work. In one study, taking 0.5 milligram of immediate-release melatonin 4 hours after bedtime (or 0.5 milligram of control-release melatonin 30 minutes before bedtime) helped people wake up about 30 minutes later, but that wasn't considered a major achievement by the researchers.

The therapy. Try a bright-light treatment in the evening between 7:00 and 9:00. Do your best to stay awake at least until 10:00, and follow our sleep hygiene suggestions.

When Cycles Attack Your Sleep

Since anything that hampers your sleep also hampers your stick-to-itiveness in the Belly Melt Diet program, we'll address how to foil the sleep problems that come with your cycles, from PMS to menopause. Getting the sleep you need will ensure that you have the strength you need (and the hormonal balance you require) to stay the course.

Placating PMS

To the list of concerns (a snoring husband, sleepless toddlers, global warming, the national debt) that keep you staring at the ceiling all night, add these two: PMS and PMDD. Premenstrual syndrome and its evil, rarer cousin, premenstrual dysphoric disorder, are products of your menstrual cycle. Symptoms—which you're likely to be up close and personal with—can range from barely noticeable to life-altering (in the case of PMDD). Bloating, edginess, fatigue, mood swings, depression, aches, pains, acne, and breast tenderness—some 85 percent of women who menstruate are prone to experiencing one or more of these every single month. More severe problems, including anxiety, major depression, food cravings, bingeing, out-of-control anger, and panic attacks may trouble the 3 to 8 percent of menstruating women who have PMDD.

The symptom that's common to both PMS and PMDD is insomnia. And cycle-triggered insomnia has a hormonal connection. For starters, melatonin (the you-are-getting-sleepy hormone) is intricately connected with your reproductive hormones. In fact, the same area of the brain houses receptors for the female hormones and for melatonin. And to digress a second, here's a piece of chemical complexity that fascinates cancer researchers: Melatonin seems to blunt the growth of estrogen receptor-alpha-positive breast cancer cells.

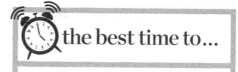

the best time to...

GET A PAP TEST

Around the time a woman is ovulating, cervical mucus is thinner, allowing for a better sampling of cells, so it's the optimal time for a Pap test. For most women, ovulation occurs in the middle of the menstrual cycle. And the best time to **Get a Mammogram:** For premenopausal women, the American Cancer Society recommends not scheduling the test the week before your period because your breasts may be swollen and tender. Most experts agree that the week after your period is the best for a mammogram, in terms of both comfort and getting the most accurate image.

The interplay between female hormones and melatonin isn't completely understood, but we do know this much—estrogen seems to reduce melatonin's sleep-inducing action, according to Robert J. Hedaya, MD, clinical professor of psychiatry at Georgetown University, writing in his blog for *Psychology Today.*

Estrogen levels go up at different times of your menstrual cycle. And, says Dr. Hedaya, there's more. Women with PMS have lower levels of progesterone toward the end of their cycles. This matters because progesterone is a reproductive hormone with a sleep-inducing side effect.

But you don't have to put up with sleepless nights month after month, he says. Happily, cycle-connected insomnia generally responds to treatment.

But first, you have to make like a detective—a very patient one—to figure out whether your hormones are to blame. Here's how:

Journal it. Track your menstrual cycle, moods, and sleep habits like a hawk for 3 months. Write down your symptoms, the time of day you noticed them, and pertinent info about your meals, snacks, and exercise.

See your gyno. Ask her about having your hormones measured at several times during your cycle to see whether their levels could be affecting your sleep. If it turns out that you have an excess of estrogen or a progesterone deficiency, for example, your doc might recommend taking supplementary progesterone. And if your melatonin levels aren't up to par, taking a melatonin supplement could help you sleep better.

Lighten up. Light therapy may help some women sleep better—especially for those whose PMS seems to worsen in the winter. According to Martha Howard, MD, an integrative practitioner and medical director of Wellness Associates in Chicago, using a light box in the late afternoon around sunset—you can put it on your desk at work—can help by simulating the effects of sunlight and lengthening the day.

Eat away symptoms. Check out our PMS-fighting foods in Chapter 6. One study found that women who got more foods with B vitamins in their diets (and not through supplements, interestingly enough) experienced fewer PMS symptoms, such as bloating, which can also keep you awake at night.

Hot Flashes, Night Sweats, and the Blues: It's Menopause

If you're a woman of a certain age—on the north side of 45, say—it may be dawning on you that you're no longer sleeping the way you used to a decade or so ago. And sleep isn't the only thing that's different about you these days, is it? Slowly creeping up on you are the symptoms—and we don't want to put too fine a point on it—that you may have been dreading. You know what we're talking about: mood swings, weight gain (especially in the belly), hot flashes and soaked sheets, and, yes, the intermittent sleep that comes with the onset of menopause.

And then there's this: Some 10 percent of women will experience major depression during menopause, and researchers aren't quite sure why. They call it the domino hypothesis, meaning that hot flashes and night sweats ruin sleep, which in turn leads to mood changes like depression. But studies haven't proven the connection. What we do know is this: Many women tangle with depression from mild to severe as they go through menopause, and depression leads to weight gain.

We urge you to embrace this time of life because it's far healthier emotionally to embrace your good life and appreciate the good years ahead than to mourn their passage. Still, despite the wisdom that comes with the advent of menopause, other changes like losing sleep and waking up at 3:00 in the morning feeling like the fire department just hosed you down are decidedly unwelcome.

In a 2005 study of 630 premenopausal women ages 43 to 53, 74 percent said they had trouble sleeping on at least one night during the month-long study, while 20 percent said they had sleeping problems 40 percent of the time. On average, the women said they slept poorly three nights a week. Among older women, as many as 61 percent of postmenopausal women report sleeping woes.

the best time to...

AVOID A HEART ATTACK

Well, that would be all the time, but in fact heart attacks happen most frequently in the morning, especially on Mondays, and are more deadly in winter, even in places where the climate doesn't change. One study found that heart attacks were three times more likely to happen between 9:00 and 10:00 a.m. than in the hour before midnight. Scientists theorize that the increase in blood pressure upon awakening may cause plaque deposits to break free. In addition, platelets—cell fragments in the blood—are stickier in the morning, and therefore more likely to create clots. What can you do? If you're at risk, move into your day slowly and deliberately, and exercise (it can reduce your risk of a heart attack by 40 percent), but don't do it first thing.

Why do so many women become raging insomniacs before, during, and after menopause? There's the obvious, of course, which is that it's pretty hard to sleep well when night sweats turn you, your pj's, and your bedding into a soggy mess. But night sweats are only part of the problem. In addition to them, menopause researchers cite other issues, including headaches, dizziness, palpitations, depression, and weight gain as reasons middle-aged women are so sleep-challenged.

You might blame it on your hormones. The older you get, the less melatonin you produce (remember, it's the hormone that makes you sleepy), which makes it harder and harder for you to fall asleep. Then, during perimenopause, which typically begins in your forties and lasts until your period finally ceases in your mid-fifties or so, your estrogen and progesterone levels bounce around. This deals a double whammy to sound sleep: When these hormone levels surge and dip, hot flashes and night sweats can ensue. And progesterone and estrogen can also help—or hurt—your ability to sleep.

Even after menopause, sleep problems continue and may even worsen. Some older women, for example, begin to produce less thyroid hormone and develop hypothyroidism. This can lead to weight gain, which increases your chances of becoming a snorer and/or having sleep apnea, a problem caused by narrowed airways that disrupt your breathing while you sleep—which undermines sleep quality.

Cool Hot Flashes Naturally

Fill a 4-ounce spray bottle with pure witch hazel. Add ½ teaspoon of pure lavender essential oil. Put the bottle in a small bucket of ice, and keep it on your night table for a chilling spritz as needed during the night.

Sleeping through the Change

Assertive changes to your diet, activity level, and sleep hygiene behaviors can help you deal with sleep problems that arise as menopause approaches. But the key to your menopausal sleep strategy is to lessen sleep-disrupting hot flashes and night sweats. Here's what you need to know:

Black cohosh. Anyone who's ever read a woman's magazine knows that The Herb for menopause is black cohosh (*Actaea racemosa,* syn. *Cimicifuga racemosa*). Its storied place in American folk tradition for easing menopausal symptoms—including hot flashes, depression, and insomnia—was affirmed back in the 1980s and '90s by a slew of clinical studies in Europe. But now experts have their doubts: A few more-recent studies have shown that black cohosh may be no more effective for relieving those sleep-disrupting hot flashes than a sugar pill. Still, the American Congress of Obstetricians and Gynecologists continues to recommend using it as an alternative treatment for menopausal symptoms including sleep problems, hot flashes, anxiety, and depression, as do herbalists and herbally trained MDs the world over.

Bottom line: Black cohosh is worth a try, especially for women who need to avoid hormone therapy. Side effects can include headaches and dizziness. Rarely, black cohosh may trigger bleeding during menopause because it stimulates the ovaries. Let your doctor know about any unusual bleeding. A black cohosh preparation that's undergone clinical testing is Remifemin. You can find it at health food stores and drugstores; follow label directions.

What about soy? When Western researchers discovered that Asian women had a fraction of the menopausal symptoms that women in the West do, they logically looked to dietary differences for clues. One jumped right out: Asian women eat more soy foods than Western women do. In fact, it's estimated that women who eat a traditional Asian diet are likely to consume between 40 and 80 milligrams of isoflavones (the active ingredient in soy) a day. In the West we eat fewer than 3 milligrams a day.

Before you could say *edamame,* soy got tagged as a major player in the war against hot flashes and other symptoms of menopause. Part of that message was terrific, healthwise: Emulate your Asian sisters by eating less red meat and more vegetarian meals that include soy foods, because doing so may alleviate symptoms. As a bonus, you may lower your risk for heart disease, cancer, and other ailments.

But don't make the mistake of thinking that soy supplements will ease your symptoms. Researchers who reviewed alternative and complementary menopause treatments in 2010 looked at 23 studies of soy supplements. According to the researchers, the results were inconclusive.

Bottom line: Stick to whole soy foods—tofu, tempeh, soybeans, and soy milk. Eating a diet rich in plant foods and light in animal foods is what most nutritionally savvy health experts recommend.

Hormone therapy. For decades, the treatment of choice for easing menopausal symptoms was hormone therapy (HT)—studies show that it can reduce hot flashes by up to 75 percent. Many docs suggested that for middle-aged women, HT was like sipping from the fountain of youth—not only would it chill hot flashes and improve your mood, but it could boost heart health, strengthen bones, and maybe even smooth out wrinkles. That was then.

Here's what we know now: Healthy women who take combination HT (progestin with estrogen, made from the urine of pregnant mares) are at a slightly increased risk for heart disease. In fact, a woman's risk of heart disease more than doubles within the first 2 years of taking a drug like Premarin. But if you do the math, you'll realize that "twice the risk" is actually a pretty small number. In the now-famous Women's Health Initiative study, which was halted in 2002 (after an average of 5.6 years of treatment), when researchers discovered the HT–heart disease connection, 8,506 women took the estrogen-plus-progestin pills. Of those, 188 women developed heart disease—80 of whom became ill within the first 2 years of therapy. In the placebo group of 8,102 women, 147 women developed heart disease, 51 within 2 years.

Bottom line: If you have disruptive hot flashes or night sweats, HT might be your ticket to better sleep during menopause. But it's not the answer for every woman. You're probably not an HT candidate if you've had breast or endometrial cancer, bouts of abnormal vaginal bleeding, or have a history of blood clots, heart disease, stroke, liver disease, or if you're pregnant or planning to become pregnant. Talk to your doctor about HT's risks and benefits.

Acupuncture. Its solid research cred makes acupuncture a good choice for women whose sleep is disrupted by hot flashes. In a 2004 Swedish study, acupuncture slashed the frequency of hot flashes by nearly half. More recently, a study by researchers at Stanford and Harvard University Schools of Medicine compared the effects of real and fake acupuncture on nighttime hot flashes. Women had two 20-minute treatments a week for 2 weeks, then weekly treatments for 5 weeks. The real acupuncture reduced nightly hot flashes by almost 30 percent; the fake treatment reduced them by 6 percent. Finally, in 2010, South Korean researchers found that three acupuncture treatments a week for a month reduced hot flash symptoms (as scored on a standardized test) by 62 percent. Women in the study's placebo group posted hot flash reductions of 27 percent.

Bottom line: Acupuncture is a safe therapy that eases hot flashes for many women. The downside is that it can be expensive—treatments can cost from $50 to upwards of $120, depending on the practitioner you choose. Some insurance companies may cover the cost for acupuncture. You can find a therapist at the American Association for Acupuncture and Oriental Medicine at www.aaaomonline.org. Click on the "patient" tab on the home page. Do make sure he or she has a state license or national board certification.

My Belly Melt

"I've lost 10 pounds, and everything feels looser."

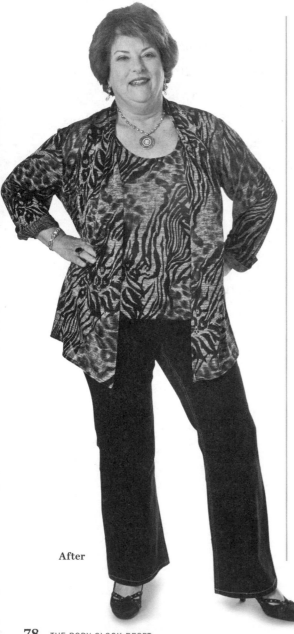

After

Lynn Jacobs

AGE: 62

POUNDS LOST: 10.2 in 35 days

POUNDS LOST IN 3-DAY RESET: 4.8

ALLOVER INCHES LOST: 5.25

INCHES FROM WAIST LOST: 2.5

BODY FAT LOST: 4.4 percent

"Last week I started noticing that everything feels looser," Lynn says. No wonder: In just 5 weeks, she lost more than 10 pounds. Her energy and self-confidence are zooming, and she forecasts clear sailing ahead. She's sleeping longer and exercising regularly. "The program changed my behavior and got me into the right mode," she explains. "I feel much better, and I want to continue.

Success Story

"I had a lot of weight to lose," Lynn adds. "I was already overweight, then I gained 20 pounds last year after I got hurt playing tennis." During the 12 months that her Achilles tendon was healing, she couldn't wear flat shoes—"not even sneakers to take a walk."

Getting into a new rhythm with the BMD Reset plan was a snap, she says. She rode a stationary bicycle every morning at home. "I was just about to leave it at the curb, because nobody was using it," Lynn recalls with a laugh. She also went to the gym a couple of times a week for circuit training, took Zumba classes twice a week, and soon was back on the tennis court.

A chronic insomniac— "Having kids destroys your sleep"—Lynn says she can't remember the last time she slept through the night. Once on the program, she started going to bed earlier—at 9:30 instead of 11:00—and getting up consistently at 6:30 a.m. She still wakes up several times during the night, but in the morning she feels more energetic and refreshed, she says.

She overhauled her diet, fine-tuning the program to suit her tastes. "I like fruit, so I'd substitute a pear or some blueberries for a salad." For a satisfying midmorning snack, she'd have a clementine and a piece of Laughing Cow low-fat cheese.

Lynn says she was surprised to find that on the program she no longer craves sweets: "I didn't have much trouble resisting desserts, which I always want." And when her daughter came to visit and brought a big bar of dark chocolate, Lynn just had a bite. "There will always be times of temptation," she notes. But she's ready now. "We were at a wedding last weekend, and I just tasted the dessert."

Before

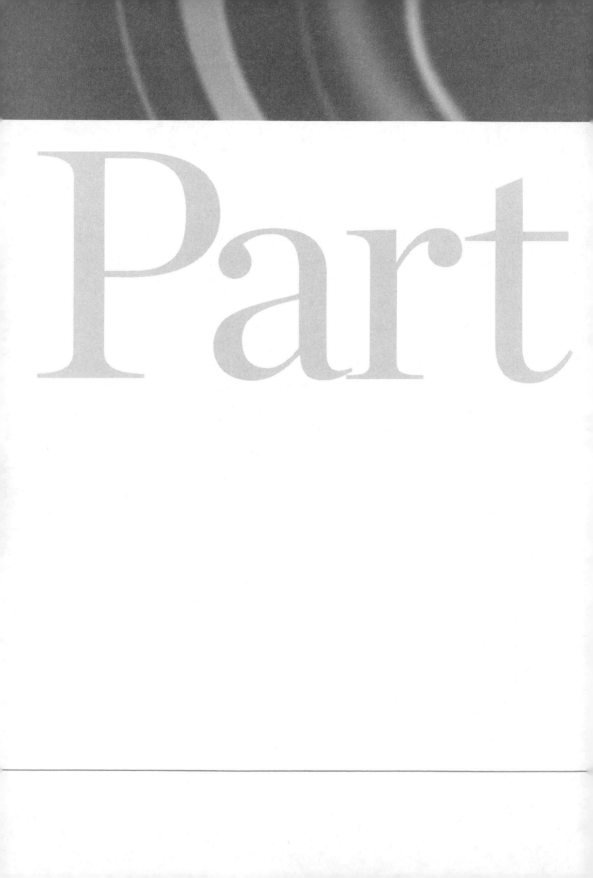

Part

II

Eat Around the Clock

Reset Your Appetite

Think about all the times you've lost and then gained weight, and how you did it. You probably did some cut-out-something-completely diet, such as fat (the low-fat craze), carbs (the Atkins craze), or meat protein (the vegan craze). Or you subscribed to some overpriced, overprocessed food-in-a-box-delivered-to-your-door-type program. And you probably reduced your calorie levels immensely, skipped meals, and cut back on snacks. Sure, you lost some weight, and it worked for a while. But eventually your body started to crave the lost calories or nutrients or the best time to...

TAKE YOUR VITAMINS

"Vitamins A, D, E, and K are fat soluble, which means they're best absorbed in the presence of fat, so they're best taken with food," says John A. Rumberger, MD, PhD, director of cardiac imaging at the Princeton Longevity Center in New Jersey. "For other, water-soluble vitamins, this doesn't matter." Since multivitamins contain fat solubles, take them with a meal. Dr. Rumberger also recommends splitting the dose, and taking vitamins twice a day to boost absorption.

real food, and so you succumbed, the weight crept back—and then you got down on yourself for another failed diet attempt.

But here's the catch: All of those actions threw a wrench into your body's natural food cycle. It wasn't that you didn't have the willpower to avoid those foods; it was that your body was operating on an inherent cycle that made you *need* those foods—so once again, you were butting heads with your body's own natural rhythms. We've said it before, and we'll say it again—you can't fight your body and win.

In the previous section, you learned how your circadian rhythm and a lack of sleep can really mess with your hunger hormones, triggering the release of ghrelin, the hunger-havoc hormone, and stagnating the release of leptin, the "I'm full" hormone. But those hunger hormones also work on their own cycles, and what you eat—and just as important, when you eat—is vital to keeping cravings at bay so that you're able to lose weight without feeling ravenous.

We've devised the Belly Melt Diet specifically to work with your body's need for certain nutrients at certain times, so that you can both enjoy your meals and head off hunger attacks before they happen. But before we get into the nuts and bolts, let's look at exactly how your body's food clock works.

Set Your Eating Schedule

As we've already seen, each of us carries the equivalent of London's Big Ben in our heads, a master clock that's keyed to light and dark cycles and tells us when to wake, when to sleep, when to eat. But even if you live in London, you're not always in sight of the huge clock at Westminster Palace. You're far more likely to keep time by your watch, your cell phone, or the wall clock in your office. Your appetite is like that, too. When it comes to eating, each of us has a set of smaller clocks in our tissues and organs and a separate food clock in the hypothalamus that act as energy sensors that tell us—with stomach rumblings and antsy feelings around mealtimes that it's time to refuel. Think of it as an invisible gas gauge that alerts us chemically when we're running on empty.

In reality, it's a complex piece of biochemical orchestration involving genes, enzymes, hormones, brain messengers, and communication molecules called neuropeptides that can be thrown into disarray by any number of things.

As you read before, a bad night's sleep alters the delicate balance of your appetite hormones, so you get more "eat" signals than "stop eating" signals. A study at the University of Chicago that was published in 2009 in the *American Journal of Clinical Nutrition* found that people who were awakened after only 5½ hours of sleep snacked 50 percent more the next day than they did when they slept 2½ hours longer. And they didn't eat less at meals to compensate for the extra nibble calories, either. (See "Why You Can't Beat the Clock: Sleep and Your Appetite" on page 96 to read more about sleep and food cravings.)

It's not just sleep that can interrupt the dance between ghrelin and leptin, the yin and yang of hunger and satisfaction. If you skip a meal, or if you have a feast one day and a pauper's meal the next, those hormones start waxing and waning, sending you hunger signals that are impossible to

A REASON FOR MENOPAUSAL MUNCHIES

Studies at Yale University found that leptin, the hormone that tells you you've had enough to eat, has a friend in estrogen, and uses the same chemical pathways to curb appetite. But once estrogen production drops, as it does after menopause, leptin may not be strong enough to fend off hunger pangs all on its own. This lack of estrogen may be the reason for the 12 percent increase in midlife weight problems in women, as compared with women in their twenties and thirties. In studies of monkeys, when their reproductive hormones plummeted, their appetites soared—they ate 67 percent more than before and gained 5 percent in body weight. That's why it's more important than ever during this time of life to quell ghrelin and its fellow hunger hormones, which is exactly what the Belly Melt Diet does.

ignore. (Ever eat almost nothing all day because you didn't feel hungry and then scarf down everything you could get your hands on that night? Yeah, that's ghrelin working.)

And then we get back to the food-entrained oscillator, or FEO, that we learned about in Chapter 1. That internal clock is triggered by sight, and was cued back in famine times to make you want food just because you saw it (since you were never sure that you'd be eating again anytime soon). But the FEO hasn't adapted to the current-day McDonald's on every street corner and Cinnabon in every mall, so the constant influx of food images disrupts your internal clock as well. In a finding that's been shown over and over again in many studies, overweight people exposed to pictures of food have a craving for the food, even if they've just eaten a filling meal.

Quiet Those Hunger Hormones

On any given day, you could be assaulted by more shouting voices in your hunger center than a trader in the commodities market pit. No wonder you've been struggling with your weight. But you can get those voices down to a dull roar—and even eliminate them completely—if you take control of just one thing: meal timing. While light and dark are powerful zeitgebers controlled by the suprachiasmatic nucleus, or SCN, you can also synchronize your body to mealtimes—in fact, to your eating behavior. (In some cases, such as jet lag, new research suggests that you can use your mealtime clock to reset your SCN to a new time zone!)

It all starts in the cradle. Think about babies. Oblivious to the 24-hour light/dark cycle, a newborn will wake up at 2:00 a.m., and again at 4:00 a.m., looking for a meal. Over time—and when more substantial food is introduced— she no longer needs those frequent postmidnight meals, but you can't always count on your infant sleeping through because she's grown accustomed to eating twice a night. A few (terrible) nights and lots of crying later (you and your baby), and you can eliminate those night feedings.

That meal-entrained clock also explains why, if you eat breakfast every morning at 8:00, you're hungry for breakfast every morning at 8:00. It's also one of the reasons you head to the vending machines for a candy bar at 3:00 every afternoon, and why the week after Christmas you're still mentally— and physically—looking for those luscious candies and yummy cookies that became a staple at the office during the holiday season. It's as if your body takes your eating habits and makes them a standing appointment, rearranging the production of appetite chemicals to suit food availability.

And, scientifically speaking, that's exactly what it does. In animal studies, rats—who can't tell time—nevertheless start exhibiting "food anticipatory behavior," such as lingering near their feeders at the time their chow is served every day. Studies in both rats and humans have found that ghrelin, the appetite-stimulating hormone, never forgets: It's set by mealtime. In one study published in 2007, researchers at Purdue University put one group of adults on an eating schedule in which there were 2½ to 3½ hours between breakfast and lunch, and another group on a tougher schedule: They had to wait 5½ to 6½ hours between the two meals. After 2 days, the researchers tested the participants' blood and found that ghrelin had risen at the specific mealtimes of each group, suggesting that the hormone likes you to eat on schedule. So while you may forget to eat, ghrelin doesn't—which is why starving yourself or skipping meals to lose weight almost always backfires.

Timing appears to be just about everything, especially when it comes to weight gain. For example, in studies by Fred Turek, PhD, director of Northwestern University's Center for Sleep and Circadian Biology in Evanston, Illinois, rats that were fed a high-fat diet at a time when they typically would have been sleeping gained weight within just 2 hours. Rats consuming the same diet during their normal awake time also gained weight—but it took them 3 weeks on the same diet to pile it on. It wasn't just when they ate but what they ate: A high-fat diet actually alters the expression of clock genes in the brain, liver, and fat tissue, Dr. Turek's group found.

And it's not only rats that struggle with timing-induced weight problems. In a now landmark study on humans by the father of chronobiology, Franz Halberg, PhD, volunteers at the University of Minnesota consumed 2,000 calories a day. During one part of the study, they consumed all 2,000 calories in the morning, and lost weight. During another part of the study, they consumed all 2,000 calories at night, and gained weight. The same 2,000 calories but eaten at different times.

So *when* you eat makes a difference in your weight, but possibly more crucial is that, by conditioning your body to eat at specific times—and eating more frequently—you can train it to expect food only at those times, thereby heading off any time-driven cravings at the pass.

Also, by eating meals and snacks at the same time—and not skipping *any* meals—you keep those hunger hormones at a steady level. Whether you feel it or not, when you skip a meal, the hormone ghrelin is building and building. You may not notice him right away, but—WHAM—before you know it, you're searching in every nook and cranny for something, *anything,* to eat. And as we said before, if you don't eat much during the day and then gorge at night (the hallmark of many a dieter), you're more likely to gain weight, since you're getting more of your calories at night.

It comes down to this: Timed eating keeps hunger hormones in check and conditions your body to eat only when it needs to—and when you're prepared to feed it with the most healthful, most satisfying fuel.

the best time to...

TAKE ASPIRIN

All findings point to late evening. In research conducted in Spain, people with pre-hypertension (borderline high) who took aspirin at 11:00 p.m. had lower blood pressure readings after 3 months than those who took it at 8:00 a.m. A study published in *Chronobiology International* found that taking aspirin at 10:00 at night produced half as many sores in the stomach lining as it did when it was taken at 10:00 in the morning.

Please Feed the Hormones

The other element of most diets that sends our body clocks into a tailspin is the rejection of certain food categories, such as carbs, fat, or protein. Those hunger hormones respond differently to different foods, and if you cut out, say, carbs, they won't be satisfied—no matter how much you eat of other foods.

Take our friend ghrelin again. It's calmed best by a combination of carbs and protein. If you're on a no-carb diet, ghrelin won't be satisfied, and it will rear its ugly head sooner than it would if you had fed it a single slice of whole wheat toast.

So now you can see another reason that other diets have failed you: Eliminating a food group left your hunger hormones out of whack—and left you open for killer hunger pangs that you just couldn't resist.

My Belly Melt

"I have so much energy, it's unbelievable!"

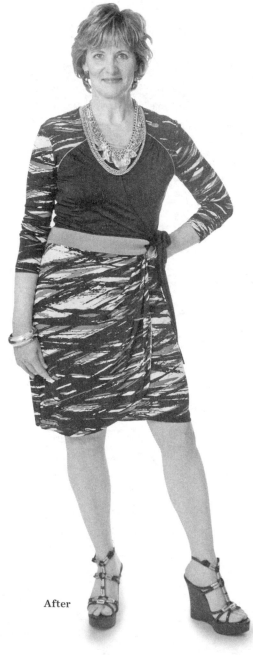

After

Lisamarie Valla

AGE: 48

POUNDS LOST: 11.6 in 35 days

POUNDS LOST IN 3-DAY RESET: 3

ALLOVER INCHES LOST: 9.5

INCHES FROM WAIST LOST: 4

BODY FAT LOST: 3.8 percent

"My husband said to me, 'Who are you, and what have you done with my wife?'" Lisamarie says, throwing back her head and laughing. "I still can't believe the changes in me and my body, and I'm thrilled with the results. I feel like I am who I was meant to be."

Lisamarie's feeling frisky because she lost nearly 12 pounds of stubborn winter weight that she put on a couple of years ago. The exercise program has ramped up her energy 24/7, she says, so much so that she'll dive in to cleaning the house in the evening after a full day at the office.

She and her guy are both delighted not only with her new shape but with her new

Success Story

focus on food planning and health. "I joined the program hoping to lose 15 pounds." She pauses and shakes her head. "Nothing else ever worked. I'd make a little headway, then fall back." For Lisamarie, the comprehensive program was the key. "I had to change how I do everything, from having the right food in the house to the way I think about eating. Now I'm fueling my body, not gorging myself." The BMD method cut her cravings and stopped her stress eating.

"I enjoy eating clean," she says. "I think it really helped my tastebuds to appreciate food more, by eliminating processed foods and thinking about the fresh/unprocessed value of everything I was making or buying. I realized how much more I was enjoying the taste of fresh food when, on day two or three, I ate a piece of plain whole wheat bread and it tasted like candy to me."

The office candy jar used to be her downfall. "I'd walk by and mindlessly grab a piece. I still see the candy there, but after the second day of the program, I didn't want it anymore."

She did reward herself with little extras from time to time—the occasional glass of wine with dinner, or a few bites of the chicken enchiladas she was fixing for her family. "The secret is being flexible but not *too* flexible," she explains. "My kids asked me if we'll ever have pizza again. Yes, we will, because now I can eat just one slice with a salad."

Lisamarie credits the BMD exercise program with lifting her energy to a 10 out of 10. "I used to fancy myself an exercise person, but I really only worked out a day or two a week. Now I really am a workout queen." Strength training in the afternoon was new, and it paid big dividends. "I'd start dinner, then do my exercises. I had so much energy, I'd clean the house after dinner. That energy from my workout carried through the whole day."

Her goal weight is in sight, and she has no intention of returning to her old ways. "This is not a crash diet; it's a lifestyle I can stick with," she says. "I just bought size 8 pants!"

Before

Timing It Perfectly

To get a better idea of how timing can affect your hunger hormones, here's a breakdown of what's going on with your food body clock throughout the day.

Early morning. The alarm clock has stirred more than you—it woke up ghrelin, the "feed me" hormone that's made in your stomach. Ignore ghrelin and not only do you set the stage for cravings later on (he just keeps getting angrier if you don't feed him), but skipping breakfast sends your natural cycle into a hormonal tailspin. Ghrelin has also nudged awake neuropeptide Y (NPY), a gut hormone that regulates appetite and the craving for carbohydrates. If you don't satisfy NPY, it will just keep building and building.

A small serving of healthy carbs—such as the vegetables in your omelet or whole wheat toast—will keep NPY from nagging you all morning and triggering those 10:00 doughnut cravings. So within the hour of waking up, treat yourself to a relatively big breakfast that mixes complex carbs (like whole grain bread or cereal) and protein (eggs, egg whites, fat-free milk, low-fat cheese). The whole grains and protein slow your blood sugar's rise and suppress ghrelin longer. And why a big breakfast? Because the food you eat in the morning has a higher satiety level—meaning it makes you feel fuller—than the food you eat at night.

After you eat (at any time of the day), levels of leptin—the appetite-suppressing hormone made by your fat cells—go up, and that tells NPY to simmer down. And as food is digested in your gut, your body produces the chemical cholecystokinin (CCK), which acts synergistically with leptin to turn off your appetite and tell you you're full.

Midmorning. Ghrelin begins to rise a couple of hours before lunch to remind you to eat. In animal studies, mice and rats start exhibiting "food anticipatory behavior," such as running in their wheels and checking the food dispenser, when the ghrelin starts pumping. Humans usually find themselves wandering to the vending machines. (See, we told you those

Eat Every 4 Hours

Don't let more than 4 hours go by without eating. Eating even "a little something" stimulates the secretion of a hormone called peptide YY-36, which reduces ghrelin production and shuts off your appetite. Also, never eat a carb without a protein. Protein slows digestion and helps keep blood sugar stable, so you'll feel full and satisfied, and fatigue won't make you succumb to bad-for-you goodies.

cravings weren't your fault!) Ghrelin turns off when you eat—particularly carbs and protein—so it's smart to have a small combo snack now. Carbs shut off ghrelin pretty quickly, and protein keeps it turned off longer. Since everyone has a different schedule, it's best to time this snack at the midpoint between your breakfast and lunch. (So if you ate breakfast at 8:00, and you plan to lunch at noon, snack at 10:00.)

Lunch. Your friend ghrelin is up again, but so is a new hunger hormone—galanin. Galanin makes you want to eat fat, and starts up at lunchtime, and peaks in the evening. However, eating a high-fat lunch isn't a good idea. Fatty foods don't suppress the "eat more" effects of ghrelin as well as carbs and proteins do (actually, hardly at all). Plus, dietary fat causes you to produce more galanin, which then tells you to eat more fat, and a vicious cycle begins. (Now you know why you can chow down an entire fatty take-out meal even after you've hit caloric overload.)

This is no time to have that big bowl of pasta, either. Carbohydrates produce a huge blood sugar spike that's followed by a precipitous drop, which can leave you tired and hungry by midafternoon. They also raise levels of the amino acid tryptophan. The body uses it to make melatonin, the sleep hormone. Ghrelin will shut off when you eat, and leptin goes up. But you'll feel fullest and most alert if you have a lunch of carbs and protein together.

The key to lunch isn't just what you eat but when—eating at the same time every day. As you can see from this complex dance of hormones, working through the lunch hour, only to wolf down something at 3:00 p.m., sends them into a tizzy, which subsequently throws your circadian cycle out of whack, as well as your body's natural hunger cycle, for the rest of the day.

Midafternoon. Time for another protein snack, like a turkey roll-up or string cheese. The amino acid tyrosine, found in protein, promotes alertness, making that your best midafternoon pick-me-up. (By the way, that slump is not in your head. It's at this point that your body temperature drops, as does blood sugar, triggered by insulin secretion after your lunch. Leptin also hits bottom. That's why you can't stop thinking about Ho Hos.) Protein also raises levels of the brain chemical dopamine, which is in charge of pleasure, as well as norepinephrine, an adrenal hormone secreted to give you sudden energy when you're under stress. It's a little like your body's own shot of espresso, making you feel perky again. Speaking of coffee, if you really need a quick blast of alertness, now's the last time to do it. Coffee after 4:00 p.m. has been shown to foil your circadian rhythms and may keep you from falling asleep tonight.

Early evening. Your body is producing ghrelin and galanin again. Ghrelin is telling you to eat, and galanin is urging you to eat fat because it wants to make sure you have enough calories on board so you don't wake up at night.

Have Your Cocktail with Dinner

Dinner is the ideal time to have a glass of wine. It gives your body enough time to metabolize the alcohol before you go into your sleep cycle. While alcohol makes you sleepy, drinking it too close to bedtime can skew brain patterns, delay dream (REM) sleep, and wake you up frequently during the night.

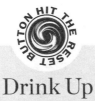

Drink Up

Another way to thwart those hunger hormones? Before every meal drink two 8-ounce glasses of water. A study from Boston University presented at the National Meeting of the American Chemical Society found that people who drank this amount before breakfast, lunch, and dinner during a 12-week program lost 5 pounds more than those who didn't chug the H_2O before meals. Previous studies have shown that people will eat up to 90 fewer calories per meal if they drink a glass of water first. Experts believe that the water fills your stomach, making you feel full. In fact, anytime you feel a craving coming on, reach for the water bottle. Thirst is often confused with hunger.

This is a great time to load up on healthy fats like olive oil and fish (which, as you'll see on page 104 is one of our Sleep and Sleek foods, because it promotes sleep and resets your body's rhythm on its own). While we want you to eat enough to stay asleep, don't overdo it: Studies show increased weight loss when you consume more of your calories in the a.m. than in the p.m. And eating at night throws off circadian rhythms.

Late evening/bedtime. You can have a small carbohydrate-rich snack at least an hour or two before bed. (Our panelists loved a small bowl of high-fiber cereal.) Nighttime carbohydrates create tryptophan, which promotes good sleep patterns. A 2007 study published in the *American Journal of Clinical Nutrition* by researchers at the University of Sydney in Australia found that high-glycemic carbs—sweet things that raise your blood sugar—can help you fall asleep faster. That surge in tryptophan helps your brain produce serotonin, the feel-good chemical that also triggers your body to make melatonin, the sleep hormone. Overnight, your body will tap into your fat stores for fuel so you don't wake up jonesing for a midnight snack. And you have a fail-safe system on board: The appetite suppressant leptin is at its peak after midnight.

WHY YOU CAN'T BEAT THE CLOCK: SLEEP AND YOUR APPETITE

You can't make up for sleep deprivation with food. Yet it's the solution your body is going to suggest when you can't take a nap. Don't listen. Here's why:

Studies in which people were deprived of 3 or 4 hours of sleep a night for a limited time have shown that there's a significant increase in snack attacks afterward. In a study at the University of Chicago, in which volunteers slept only 5½ hours a night, their snacking increased by more than 50 percent. Since those nibbles were overwhelmingly of the carbohydrate variety, it's clear that what the body looks for is quick energy to get through the day.

Here's why it ought to work: Carbs provide instant pep in the form of a flood of glucose into the bloodstream and cells. Here's why it doesn't: Those sugary highs quickly turn into sugary lows as blood sugar drops. And carbs boost your body's level of tryptophan, the raw material it uses to make the sleep hormone melatonin. So you're basically eating a sleeping pill in food form.

And even though the sleep-deprived study volunteers consumed extra calories in their frequent pick-me-ups, they didn't eat less at meals to compensate. It's easy to see why sleep deprivation can lead to excess weight, obesity, and the risk of developing metabolic syndrome and diabetes.

In some of these studies, scientists found that lack of sleep also alters the balance of leptin, the appetite suppressant, and ghrelin, the "feed me" hormone, so that your body produces the "eat" and "stop eating" signals at the wrong

You Have Plenty of Free Time

Don't worry about figuring all this out: We've done the work for you! The Belly Melt Diet will help you take control of your food clock so you're not so hungry that you eat everything in sight, you no longer crave high-fat junk food, and you feel so satisfied after a meal that you won't be prowling the kitchen 20 minutes later. You'll reset your food clock with a meal schedule that's based on timing—you have to eat three meals and two or three snacks at the same general time every day. No special prepackaged foods to buy, no weird ingredients, no giving up a favorite food forever. You'll simply eat the time—or, in some cases, the message to stop simply doesn't make it to the hypothalamus, the appetite center of the brain.

Some research suggests that a steady diet of high-carb meals and snacks can, over time, cause the cell-damaging free radical molecules—which your body produces naturally after you eat—to attack appetite-suppressing cells in the hypothalamus called POMC neurons, which contain receptors for leptin. Think of those receptors as a kind of special-ized mailbox that receives messages from certain body chemicals. If those receptor-studded cells are destroyed, even though your body may produce leptin, its "stop eating" messages won't get through to your brain, since there will be fewer places in which to deliver them.

But there's another, less scientific-sounding reason that sleep deprivation may pile on the pounds: If you're consistently getting only 6 or so hours of sleep a night, you have a few more hours of awake time to be raiding the fridge. You're also likely to be doing it at night, when you're apt to be tired, your body is prone to hanging on to calories as fat, and you're less likely to feel satisfied, no matter how much you eat.

And remember that ghrelin reappears like clockwork at your set mealtimes. So if you're chowing down seven or eight times a day just to keep up your energy, over time the hormone will synchronize with your eating habits, making you feel hungry at those seven or eight times a day.

foods you love at certain times to help you shrink that bad belly fat and lose weight for good.

And because you'll be consuming the foods your body wants at those times, you won't have a lingering yen for carbs or fat. If you eat according to your body clock—when it's reset and keeping perfect time, not desynchronized to run fast or slow—you'll be eating the kinds of foods you need at every point of the day to keep hunger at bay, reduce cravings, boost energy, and even help you sleep. And you'll lose weight. All of our test dieters did. And you know what? They weren't hungry.

WHY CAN'T I JUST TAKE LEPTIN?

It's a logical question. In 1994, when researchers discovered leptin, the hormone that tells us to stop eating, they thought at first that they'd discovered a magic pill for weight loss. Pop a little leptin every day, and cupcakes would no longer call to you.

But it didn't work out that way. Only people with a rare form of obesity caused by a mutation of the gene that regulates leptin lost weight with hormone injections.

For one thing, leptin may be little match for its opposite ghrelin, which is a persistent appetite noodge, as befits a hormone we developed as a hedge against starving to death when food was less available. As it turned out, leptin was just one of several chemicals that send messages to the hypothalamus, the brain region governing hunger and appetite that tells us to eat and to stop eating. In addition to ghrelin, which is made in the stomach, there are brain cells that produce chemicals that turn on appetite, and brain cells that churn out chemicals to turn it off.

A full belly also sends satiety messages to your brain via the vagus and other nerves in the stomach and the small intestine that are activated when your stomach and intestinal muscles stretch as they fill with food. The hormone cholecystokinin (CCK) produced by your small intestine closes off the sphincter muscle between it and your stomach. That causes your stomach to fill up faster and sends a message on the vagus nerve "wire" to your hypothalamus that basically says, "Enough already." In experiments, scientists can trigger the process by expanding a balloon in the stomach. This may be why both high-fiber foods, which tend to fill up the tummy, and protein, which delays the transfer of food into the intestines, can be a boon to dieters, helping them feel full faster and longer. (There's plenty of both in the Belly Melt Diet.)

Yet despite what seems like a fail-safe system, we can all manage to eat more when we're full, particularly if we get a look at the dessert cart. How does that happen? In 2011, University of Cincinnati researchers found that ghrelin enhances our sense of smell—and is probably what makes the scent of baking bread, sautéed onions, and apple pie so irresistible. Dieters tend to produce ghrelin like crazy—after all, dieting is a little like starvation—which is likely why it's so hard to stick to a weight-loss eating plan.

The solution? Keep that ghrelin level as under control as possible, which is exactly what the Belly Melt Diet program is all about.

Hunger vs. Appetite

While we can help you control your hunger hormones to an extent, there is an issue that plagues many women: How do you know when you're *really* hungry? Most people will say, "My stomach starts growling." Others will say, "I feel empty." Both of these are common physical reactions to being hungry. Your stomach growling is nothing more than the noise made when your muscles contract in an empty stomach. The empty feeling is caused by a drop in blood sugar. You may actually feel weak when you've waited too long between meals.

But how many times have you eaten when you're *not* hungry? Before you answer, ask yourself if you ever:

- Shared your dining companion's nachos even though you thought you really weren't hungry enough to order an appetizer yourself.
- Said yes to the molten lava cake after eating an appetizer, a plate of pasta, and a side salad—*and* unbuttoned your pants.
- Got so stressed out by the report you were trying to write that you ate an entire sleeve of cookies.
- Bought cinnamon buns while at a mall just because you smelled them baking.
- Stuck a candy bar on the conveyer belt at the grocery checkout.
- Felt restless and bored and wandered to the kitchen looking for something good to eat.
- Were so tired after a long night that your major exercise the next day was hitting the vending machines just to stay awake at your desk.

If you answered yes to any of those—and let's face it, if you've done one, you've probably done them all—you have some idea of the difference between hunger and appetite.

Most of us at some point eat when we're not really hungry. In fact, you may never let yourself get hungry. Instead, because you nosh all day long, you wouldn't know a hunger cue if it came up and bit you. "And when that's coupled with emotions, it's hard to tease out when you're really hungry," says Joan Salge Blake, RD, LDN, clinical associate professor of nutrition at Boston University and the author of *Nutrition and You: Core Concepts for Good Health*. "You may be eating because you're bored, stressed, or trying to avoid something," she explains. "You figure if you get a little snack, the monthly report you're trying to write will miraculously unfold on your computer screen. One rule of thumb is that if you ate a good, balanced breakfast and you're hungry an hour and a half later, there's a good chance you're not hungry, but you're bored or stressed or tired."

On the Belly Melt Diet, we recommend that, before you eat, you check in with your hunger cues. Listen for ghrelin telling you to eat before you take a bite. Pay attention to leptin, which may not get its "stop eating" message to your hypothalamus until after you've finished your meal. Often the hunger hormones speak far more softly than the emotional and situational reasons why we eat—and overeat—so they're easy to override.

Nutritionists have a handy little scale that can help you assess your hunger, and we've adapted it here. It allows you to rate your hunger on a scale of 1 to 10, with 1 being extremely hungry, and 10 being "can't eat another thing." Ask yourself how you feel each time you want to eat something, and while you're consuming a meal. We recommend that you wait until your hunger is at 3 or lower before eating, and between 4 and 6 while you're eating, to let you know when to stop. If you rank your hunger at 4 or higher before eating, do something else, like take a walk or drink a couple of glasses of water. We get most of the fluid we need every day via food, so it's easy to mistake thirst for hunger.

And if you discover that you're not hungry, ask yourself if you're eating for emotional reasons. If you are, look for a distraction with benefits (including keeping you away from food), such as walking, organizing family photos, knitting, doing a crossword puzzle or sudoku, or hitting the courts (or the Wii) for a rousing game of tennis.

The Hunger Scale

1. Ravenously hungry. My stomach is growling, and I think I may faint.

2. Very hungry. I need to eat soon.

3. My stomach feels empty, it's growling, and I'm getting hungry.

4. I could eat . . . or not.

5. I'm not hungry, but I'm not totally full.

6. Feelin' good—tummy is full, and I'm satisfied.

7. Almost full.

8. Really full.

9. Why didn't I wear my elastic-waist pants?

10. Why did I eat all that? I think I'm going to be sick.

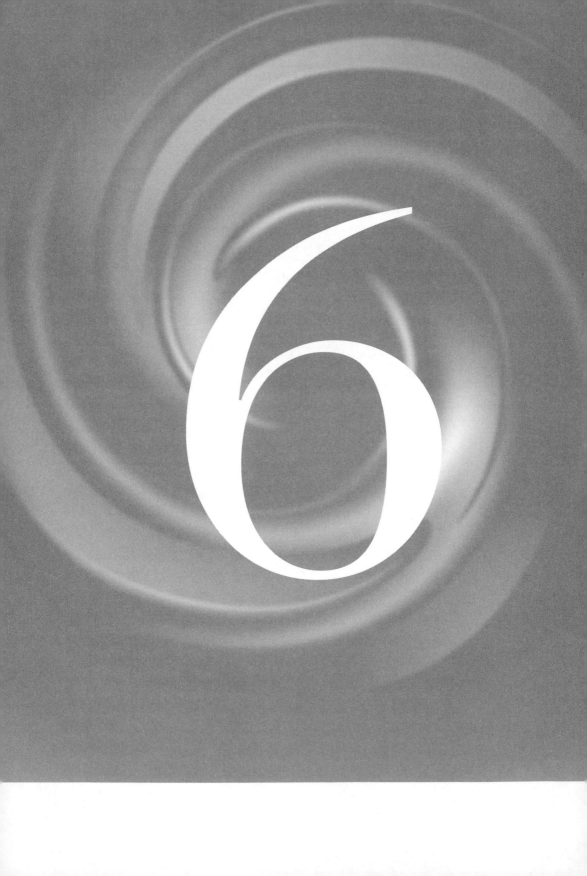

Your Sleep and Sleek Foods

So now you've learned that getting a good night's sleep will help you lose the weight you want. And you've also discovered that by eating the right foods at the right times, you can satisfy your body's need for fuel and taste, all while watching the inches slip away. Now you've come to the part where the two worlds—sleep and sleek—magically and most wonderfully collide.

There are other foods that have specific actions to help you sleep and reset your circadian rhythms. And the great news about these foods is that they also help with weight loss on their own. They provide a double shot of power to help you lose the weight you want and feel great! They're built into the Belly Melt Diet meal plans and recipes, but you can also incorporate them into your diet in any way you like. Here's a primer.

Omega-3 fatty acids. We know from animal studies that when your diet is deficient in these fats, the natural rhythms of your pineal gland—the pea-size endocrine gland in the center of your brain—are thrown off, leading to alterations in the production of melatonin, the sleep hormone. Animals with an omega-3 deficit don't sleep during their usual rest periods—they're up and spinning in their wheels the same way that humans with insomnia restlessly toss and turn. A diet rich in omega-3s is also linked to better heart health, lower risk of dementia, improved moods, and lower blood pressure.

As for weight loss, many omega-3 carriers are rich in protein. And study after study confirms: Protein makes you feel full. Your body takes longer to digest protein; it delays gastric emptying—the movement of food through your digestive system. You even burn more calories digesting protein—a process called the thermic effect of food—than you do when you eat fats or carbs. It helps slow the blood sugar spike you get from eating carbohydrates, and helps prevent the blood sugar low that usually follows. The other omega-3 superstars are fiber-rich vegetables, another set of great allies in the fight against extra fat. The best sources of Sleep and Sleek omega-3s are:

- Mackerel
- Lake trout
- Herring
- Sardines
- Albacore tuna
- Salmon
- Halibut
- Walnuts
- Flaxseed
- Dark, leafy green vegetables
- Fortified foods such as eggs, yogurt, and soy milk
- You can also supplement with fish oil capsules, flaxseed oil capsules, algae, and DHA, a component of fish oil that's available as a supplement.

Magnesium. Magnesium is a cog in the inner workings of your biological clock. Without enough magnesium in your body, your suprachiasmatic nucleus, or SCN, and pineal gland, where the sleep hormone melatonin is produced, desynchronize, which can affect your sleep as well as your mood. Research has found that people with low magnesium levels have a corresponding drop in melatonin. What we know about magnesium's effect on sleep comes from some serious sleepers. Animals who hibernate in the winter get an uptick in magnesium—sometimes two-thirds higher than normal—when they doze off. The signal to hibernate—and the rise in the magnesium—are apparently triggered by cold temperatures, suggesting that there's a seasonal variation in magnesium levels. In humans, magnesium deficiency may play a role in seasonal affective disorder (SAD), the depression and carb-craving condition brought on by the low light of winter.

A 2010 study by USDA researchers, published in *Magnesium Research,* found that magnesium supplementation can help people who have a hard time sleeping to doze peacefully through the night. One group of the 100 tossers and turners over age 51 was given 320 milligrams of magnesium a day, while the other group was given a look-alike placebo. After 7 weeks, those taking the magnesium were sleeping better, and, as a bonus, had lower levels of dangerous inflammation, a rogue reaction by the immune system that is implicated in heart disease, cancer, diabetes, and Alzheimer's disease.

A deficiency in this muscle-relaxing mineral may also be a contributing factor in PMS. In a Spanish study, women with PMS who took a timed-release supplement of 250 milligrams of magnesium experienced significant improvements in all of their symptoms. Having magnesium-rich foods always on the menu can also help you sleep if muscle soreness or cramps tend to wake you at night—the mineral, along with calcium, helps relax muscle nerves and fibers.

Once again, you'll notice that foods rich in magnesium are also extremely weight loss friendly: protein-rich fish and nuts, veggies, and fiber-rich grains. The best Sleep and Sleek foods for magnesium are:

- Halibut
- Almonds
- Cashews
- Soybeans
- Spinach
- Nuts, mixed
- Cereal, shredded wheat
- Oatmeal, instant, fortified
- Potato, baked, with skin
- Peanuts, dry roasted
- Peanut butter
- Wheat bran

- Black-eyed peas
- Yogurt, plain
- Fat-free milk
- Bran flakes
- Vegetarian baked beans
- Long-grain brown rice
- Lentils
- Avocado
- Kidney beans
- Pinto beans
- Wheat germ

Calcium. While the link between calcium and weight loss is still tenuous (in some studies it promotes greater weight loss, in others it's a wash), it turns out that milk may really do a body good when it comes to belly fat. A 2010 study by researchers at the University of Alabama at Birmingham found that, among a group of more than 100 premenopausal women, intra-abdominal fat—unceremoniously but accurately measured by X-ray absorptiometry and CAT scan—was significantly reduced in those who consumed the most calcium-rich foods. In fact, for every 100 milligrams of calcium they consumed per day (that's ½ cup of soft-serve frozen yogurt), they lost an inch of intraabdominal fat—the really bad stuff tucked in and around your internal organs that's linked to higher rates of heart disease and cancer.

The bone builder also will help you reset your menstrual cycle. To avoid PMS symptoms, including cravings, get milk. A number of studies have found that calcium from both food and supplements (in the form of carbonate) significantly reduces mood swings, carb cravings, and fatigue in women with PMS. Results from the Nurses Health Study suggest that having the equivalent of four servings a day of skim or low-fat milk, fortified orange juice, or low-fat dairy products such as yogurt, which supply 1,200 milligrams of calcium and 400 milligrams of vitamin D, protects against the monthly misery. One possible explanation: Calcium and D levels fluctuate across the menstrual cycle—an infradian rhythm—in response to female sex hormones; some studies have also found rhythmic changes in other parathyroid hormones (calcium is one) over the course of the cycle. So getting enough calcium and vitamin D helps even those out during your PMS phase.

Like magnesium, calcium can help you sleep if you tend to be awakened by muscle soreness or cramps—the mineral, along with calcium, helps relax muscle nerves and fibers. The best Sleep and Sleek sources of calcium are:

- Yogurt, plain, low-fat
- Sardines, canned in oil
- Cheddar cheese
- Milk, nonfat
- Milk, reduced-fat (2% milk fat)
- Milk, lactose-reduced
- Milk, buttermilk
- Mozzarella, part-skim
- Yogurt, fruit, low-fat
- Orange juice, calcium-fortified
- Tofu, firm, made with calcium sulfatc
- Salmon, pink, canned, solids with bone
- Pudding, chocolate, instant, made with 2% milk
- Cottage cheese, 1% milk fat
- Tofu, soft, made with calcium sulfate
- Spinach, cooked
- Ready-to-eat cereal, calcium-fortified
- Instant breakfast drink, various flavors and brands, powder prepared with water
- Frozen yogurt, vanilla, soft-serve
- Turnip greens, boiled
- Kale, cooked
- Kale, raw

Foods to Feed Your Other Cycle

Your desire to eat everything you see with chocolate on it in the week or so leading up to your period can't be explained simply by the flux of ghrelin and leptin. Most studies find ghrelin unchanged and leptin actually higher during this time, which suggests that you should have even better control of your eating behavior before your period.

But appetite is far more than the simple checks and balances of two hormones. In fact, some major researchers think that carbohydrate cravings in the luteal phase may be an attempt to self-medicate depression. Both cravings and depression are symptoms of premenstrual syndrome (PMS) and premenstrual dysphoric disorder (PMDD), a more severe form of PMS.

The link? Serotonin, the brain chemical that governs sleep and mood. Studies by Andrea Rapkin, MD, and her colleagues at the UCLA School of Medicine found marked physical differences between women with PMS and those who didn't have it. In the 10 days before getting their periods, women who had no PMS symptoms experienced a rise in levels of serotonin, the neurochemical your body uses to make the sleep hormone melatonin and that boosts your mood. Women who had PMS, on the other hand, experienced a

Whip Up a Crave-Reducing Shake

The Belly Melt Diet creator, Shari Citron, RD, came up with a satisfying, easy-to-whip-up—and did we mention delicious?—"milk shake" to treat yourself to when you feel a killer craving coming on. It's loaded with calcium, omega-3s, and protein, so you'll reset your body clock, feel full, and set yourself up for a great night's sleep—all while it helps you lose weight. You'll find the recipe on page 231.

decline in the neurotransmitter. Experiments by Barbara L. Parry, MD, at the University of California at San Diego, revealed low levels of melatonin in women with PMDD, suggesting that they too were serotonin deficient.

These days, a serotonin selective reuptake inhibitor (SSRI), the class of drugs used to treat depression, is the frontline medication for severe PMS and PMDD. But you can make serotonin yourself naturally by indulging your body's craving for carbs—not an entire pie or a candy bar but "a little something" like a low-fat biscotti, a whole wheat English muffin, or popcorn, which does double duty for PMS cravings. Carbs not only raise your serotonin levels to even out your mood, but studies by MIT's Judith Wurtman, PhD, found that carb cravings disappear when you feed them in a way that raises levels of serotonin. In one of her studies, volunteers who were given a carb drink an hour before lunch and dinner lost more weight and had less trouble sticking to their diets than women given an identical-looking drink that wasn't high in carbs. In another, women with PMS who consumed the same drink lost the mood swings and the carb cravings. (Try our Crave-Reducing Shake on page 231.)

Other studies have identified foods that cut down on PMS cravings. We mentioned above that Sleep and Sleek nutrients magnesium and calcium are wonderful PMS tamers. But a recent study has shown that B vitamins—specifically thiamin and riboflavin, found in foods such as leafy greens, fortified cereals, and nuts—are also successful in easing PMS symptoms. A study at the University of Massachusetts at Amherst looking at the diets of more than 3,000 women enrolled in the Nurses Health Study found that the more thiamin- and riboflavin-rich foods they ate, the less likely they were to experience PMS symptoms. To get this benefit, you need to consume more than the 1.1 milligrams of each vitamin recommended per day for women. Most of the PMS-free women consumed 1.9 milligrams or more. The best PMS-taming B-rich foods are:

Thiamin:

- Lentils
- Peas
- Long-grain brown rice
- Long-grain white rice, enriched
- Whole wheat bread
- Fortified breakfast cereal
- Wheat germ breakfast cereal
- Pork, lean (cooked)
- Brazil nuts
- Pecans
- Spinach
- Orange
- Cantaloupe
- Milk
- Eggs

THE "OTHER" HUNGERS

We've already brought up that killer of diets everywhere—hedonic hunger, a strong desire to eat that luscious [fill in your own favorite temptation] sitting in front of you or luring you from the kitchen. Technically, it's not hunger at all, but appetite. You may think of it as a craving—and you'd be right. If there are emotions involved—sadness, depression, anxiety, boredom—chances are what you're yearning for is something sweet. (Likewise, if it happens like clockwork in the 2 weeks before your period.) And there are two good reasons for that.

SWEET THINGS ARE NATURE'S HEROIN. Well, heroin lite. Like addictive drugs, they stimulate your body to release opioids and produce dopamine, a neurotransmitter that helps control the reward and pleasure centers of the brain. It's dopamine that drives you to do what gives you pleasure, even if it means going out in the snow for that slice of New York cheesecake you're craving. You're not technically hungry—if it were hunger, you'd be satisfied with a bowl of cereal. What you're experiencing is a strong desire for certain foods, usually something really tasty that tickles your pleasure center.

Is sugar addictive, like heroin? It looks that way in rats. In studies done at Princeton University, rats that were fed sugar water with their chow acted like a bunch of junkies going cold turkey—their teeth chattered, their forepaws trembled, and their heads shook when their sugar water was withheld. They also acted anxious and depressed. And when the sugary stuff was available again, they binged on it—not surprising, since there's evidence that ghrelin, the appetite stimulator, is also involved in cravings, particularly those that arise when stress hormones are activated.

Riboflavin:

- Fortified cereal
- Milk (nonfat)
- Cheddar cheese
- Eggs
- Almonds
- Salmon
- Halibut
- Chicken, light meat
- Chicken, dark meat
- Beef
- Broccoli
- Asparagus
- Spinach
- Bread, whole wheat

CARBS ARE NATURE'S TRANQUIL-IZERS. They're the basis of the recipe that your body uses to make you calm and relaxed. Carbs raise levels of the essential amino acid tryptophan, which has a calming influence on you (tryptophan supplements were once touted as sleep aids). Once tryptophan is in your central nervous system, it's synthesized into the brain chemical serotonin, which gives you a sense of well-being and calm. Significantly, most new antidepressants act in various ways to keep more serotonin circulating in your brain.

But while the science may make it seem like using chocolate chip cookies to boost your mood is just heeding your body's wisdom, it's really not all that smart. Sugary carbs may calm you down, but as the animal studies suggest, they also may set you up for binge eating and more cravings, which will be hard habits to break.

There's also increasing evidence, mainly from animal studies, that glucose—that's sugar to you—is a zeitgeber, a time shifter that can alter your body clock to create cravings. In one study, rats that were kept in the dark and given chocolate at the same time every day altered their behavior and activities to treat time—they displayed "food anticipatory behavior" like wheel running and lingering where the food usually appeared. It seems that once you have that sugary midafternoon snack, you think you can't live without it. Especially if your snack alarm goes off at the same time every day.

That's why the Belly Melt Diet takes all of these factors into account—it revamps your food anticipatory behavior, frees you from sugar cravings, and gives you enough carbs, protein, and fats so that your mood and hunger hormones stay under control.

My Belly Melt

"I've been set free from sugar!"

Karen Posten

AGE: 58

POUNDS LOST: 15.4 in 35 days

POUNDS LOST IN 3-DAY RESET: 3.6

ALLOVER INCHES LOST: 8.75

INCHES FROM WAIST LOST: 4.5

BODY FAT LOST: 1.5 percent

Karen Posten lost more than 15 pounds on the Belly Melt Diet—and a stellar 4½ inches from her waist—but what she's gained is just as important: the confidence that she will continue to lose weight and be able to keep it off. "I feel like I've been set free from sugar," she says. "I'm in New York City today, and I'm not craving a slice of cheesecake." For Karen, the ultimate prize is a self-sustaining healthy living plan. It shortcuts her cravings like nothing else ever has.

Karen says she's a new woman. "Emotionally, it's like night and day. Letting go of the sugar is a major plus." Her blood

After

Success Story

pressure is down 16 points to a healthy 112/78, and she says she's sleeping better than before.

She tried plenty of diets, but none of them worked for her. And now the Belly Melt Diet has made her victorious in a lifelong battle with the scale. "I'm constantly trying to lose weight. It was my struggle as a teenager. My daughter and I lost some together, but then she went to college, and I started gaining again." Now Karen and her daughter Erin (profile on page 337) are both big losers on the BMD plan.

The food allowance felt sufficient to Karen, even generous. "When I graduated to Phase 2 and could have two mini-muffins at breakfast instead of one, I thought, 'Wow, I can have this much?' I didn't always need the second."

These days, she haunts the produce aisle at the supermarket. "I don't buy packaged food anymore. I have no desire to." She knows that when she reaches her weight goal, she'll be able to stay the course: "Then I'll be able to play around with the food plan a little, as long as I stick with fresh foods and vegetables."

While Karen always knew that exercise is important, too often life got in the way. "Walking is my best exercise, but I never seemed to find the time," she explains. Now, 6 days a week, she rises and shines for an early morning walk with her friend Mary Davis (profile on page 42). And her afternoon strength training has made her stronger and cured aches and pains. "What a difference," she says. "When I started doing it, I struggled to get up off the floor. After a couple of weeks, it wasn't a problem anymore."

Sleep is a work in progress. After practicing her good-sleep routine, she says, "I still wake up at 1:00 a.m., but I'm not tossing and turning like I used to."

Karen is thrilled to be walking this path toward good health with her daughter. "When Erin started talking about summer, I was so excited that she's thinking longterm. This plan is here to stay."

Before

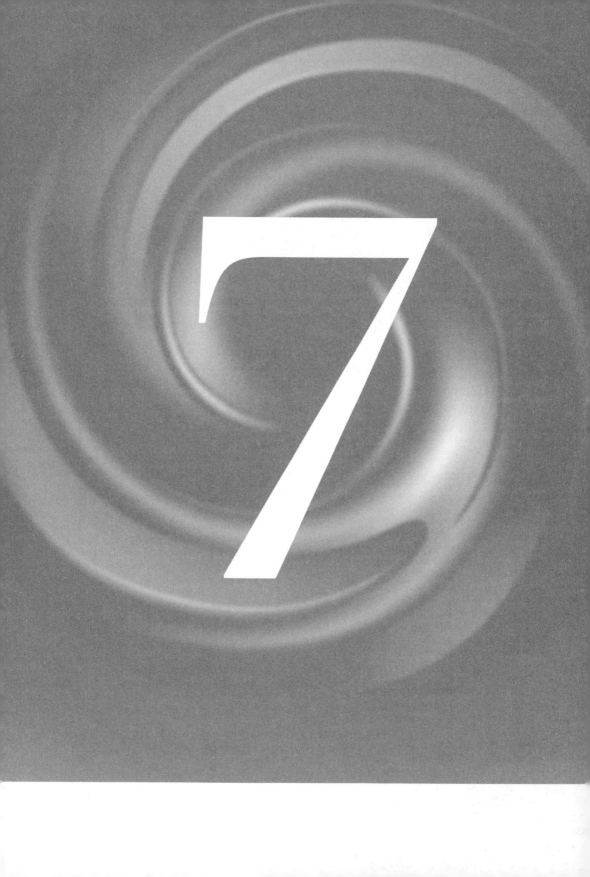

Lose Up to 8 Pounds in 3 Days

The Belly Melt Diet works to help you drop pounds by resynchronizing your circadian rhythms. Now you're ready for the all-important first phase, which we call Reset. It's a 3-day plan that should result in a quick initial weight loss—nine test panelists lost an average of almost 5 pounds in just those 3 days. The calories in this plan aren't enough to sustain you for the long run, but the elation you'll feel when the scale starts to move will give you great motivation to stick with it.

Based on everything you've read so far, this quick-start plan will reset your hunger hormones to stop cravings. First, you'll eat at specific times so that the hunger hormone ghrelin (the substance that triggers cravings and makes you want to eat) is under control at all times. Second, you'll be eating meals that provide a perfect balance of carbs, protein, and fats that will keep ghrelin under control but that will also stimulate you when you need it (during the day) and calm you when you don't (when it's time to go to sleep). Third, you'll also be choosing foods with nutrients that help you sleep better, which in turn helps reset your body clock so the weight will come off faster.

Since the plan focuses on whole, nonprocessed foods, you'll feel healthier and kick any addictions to refined sugar and additives that are also messing with your body clock. Why whole foods? It's not just because they have more nutrients—which they do—but they have other health benefits over processed foods. According to a study by researchers at Pomona College in California, people who consumed whole, unprocessed food burned more calories than those who ate processed food that had the same amount of calories. That's right, subjects who ate cheese sandwiches made with real cheese and whole grain bread burned almost 10 percent more calories than those who ate processed cheese sandwiches on white bread, thanks to an amazing little natural process we call diet-induced thermogenesis (sometimes called the thermic effect of feeding). Basically, it's the calories we burn just by digesting what we eat. Our bodies simply use up more calories when we consume whole foods. So if you're following a 1,200- to 1,500-calorie diet, as you are on the Belly Melt Diet, that means you can possibly burn an extra 120 to 225 calories each day!

The 3-day limit will snap your system back to a healthier way of eating and give you a speedy starting weight loss to encourage you to keep going, but you'll quickly move up to 1,500 calories, so there's no need to panic about feeling hungry. (That said, even in Phase 1, our panelists reported that they rarely felt hungry.)

Daily Guidelines

- 1,200 total calories
- 4 servings grains (preferably whole grain, fiber-rich)
- 2–3 servings vegetables (2–3 cups total)
- 1 serving fruit (1 cup total)
- 2–3 servings fat-free or low-fat dairy (2½ cups total)
- 3–4 servings protein (lean meat, poultry, and fish)
- 1 serving fats and oils

Meal-by-Meal Guidelines

While you are allowed flexibility on the Reset phase and don't have to follow these to a T to lose weight, this breakdown of servings has been shown to best keep hunger hormones in check and give you energy throughout the day, yet set you into a calming ready-to-sleep-off-the-pounds mode at night.

Breakfast: 1 protein, 1 grain, ½ vegetable, ½ fat

Snack: 1 dairy, ½ fruit

Lunch: 1 protein, 1½ to 2 vegetables, ½ fat

Snack: 1 dairy, ½ fruit

Dinner: 2 proteins, 2 grains, 1 vegetable

Snack: 1 grain, ½ dairy

Beverages: Drink two 8-ounce glasses of water before each meal and one before each snack.

SERVING SIZE GUIDELINES
(Each Equals 1 Serving)

GRAIN CHOICES

- 1 whole grain mini-bagel

- 1 slice whole wheat bread

- 1 small (6") whole wheat or whole grain corn tortilla

- 4 snack-size slices rye bread

- ½ whole wheat English muffin

- 1 small whole wheat muffin

- ½ cup cooked oatmeal or 1 packet instant

- 1 cup toasted oat or whole wheat flakes

- 5 whole wheat crackers or 2 rye crispbreads

- ½ cup brown wild rice, cracked wheat (bulgur) or quinoa, or cooked whole wheat pasta

VEGETABLE CHOICES (1 serving is equal to 1 cup of the following, except where noted)

- broccoli

- cauliflower

- summer squash

- carrots

- cabbage

- winter squash

- cooked beans

- tofu

- green peas

- corn (1 ear)

- tomato (1 medium)

- mashed sweet or white potatoes

- mashed pumpkin

- spinach, cooked

- collards

- mustard

- turnip

- kale

- vegetable juice

- 2 cups raw leafy greens, such as spinach, romaine, watercress, dark green leafy lettuce, endive, and escarole

FRUIT CHOICES (1 serving is equal to 1 cup of the following, except where noted)

- small apple

- medium pear

- 3 medium plums

- large orange

- medium grapefruit

- large banana

- cantaloupe

- grapes

- orange sections

- pineapple chunks

- sliced strawberries

- watermelon balls

- 100% fruit juice, such as orange, apple, grape, and grapefruit

- ½ cup dried fruit

DAIRY CHOICES

- 1 cup fat-free or low-fat milk

- 1 cup (8 ounces) fat-free or low-fat yogurt

- 1½ ounces low-fat hard cheese such as Cheddar, mozzarella, Swiss, and Parmesan

- ⅓ cup shredded cheese

- ½ cup part-skim ricotta cheese

- 2 cups low-fat cottage cheese

- 1 cup pudding made with fat-free or low-fat milk

PROTEIN CHOICES

- 1 ounce cooked fish or shellfish, lean beef, pork, ham, chicken, or turkey

- 1 whole egg

- 2 egg whites

- ½ ounce nuts (7 walnut halves, 12 almonds, 24 pistachios)

- ½ ounce seeds (pumpkin, sunflower)

- ¼ cup cooked beans (black, kidney, pinto, or white) or peas (chickpeas, lentils, or split peas)

- ¼ cup baked or refried beans

- ¼ cup (2 ounces) tofu

- 1 ounce tempeh

- ¼ cup roasted soybeans

- 1 falafel patty

- 2 tablespoons hummus

- 1 tablespoon peanut or almond butter

FAT CHOICES

- 1 teaspoon vegetable oil

- 1 tablespoon low-fat mayonnaise

- 2 tablespoons light salad dressing

- 1 tablespoon regular salad dressing

- 1 teaspoon butter

When Cravings Hit, Take a Walk

Even if your willpower is severely tested—there's a candy bar on the kitchen counter—you can successfully resist if you hoof it. Scientists at the University of Exeter in England tested the theory on a group of chocoholics and found that even when they were stressed out (the researchers tossed some mental challenges their way) and were forced to unwrap a chocolate bar, the walk made their cravings disappear. Don't have time for a stroll around the office? Try to wait it out, with the object of your desire nowhere in sight. Most cravings last only about 10 minutes, experts say, so anything you can do to distract yourself for a little while will help.

Reset 3-Day Meal Plan

Now you can always make your own meals and snacks based on what we've given you, but if you'd like some more delicious and creative ways you can eat on the BMD program, follow this 3-day meal plan created by our registered dietitian Shari Citron. Using all the studies and information we know about leptin, ghrelin, and the need to time your meals and have a perfect mix of carbs, proteins, and fats, Shari created 3 days' worth of tastebud-pleasing meals. Feel free to follow exactly, mix and match between days, or use some and then create your own using the guidelines on page 118 for others.

(*Note:* Most meals adhere to the meal-by-meal guidelines, although a few take a serving from one meal or snack and add it to another. You'll see these marked throughout.)

Day 1

Breakfast
Garlic 'n' Herb Vegetable Egg Scramble (page 149)

(uses ½ extra dairy)

Midmorning Snack
½ cup orange sections

¾ ounce fat-free hard cheese

(omits ½ dairy)

Lunch
Edamame Salad with Carrot Ginger Dressing (page 166)

Carrot Ginger Dressing (page 166)

Midafternoon Snack
Crave-Reducing Shake (page 231)

Dinner
Toasted Quinoa with Shrimp, Grapefruit, and Vegetables (page 213), served with your choice of ½ grain

Evening Snack
1 cup ready-to-eat bran flakes cereal with ½ cup nonfat milk

Per day: 1,210 calories, 80 g protein, 170 g carbohydrates, 27 g total fat, 7 g saturated fat, 29 g fiber, 2,240 mg sodium

Day 2

Breakfast

Savory Apricot-Stuffed French Toast with Tomatoes (page 150)

Midmorning Snack

1 cup 0% plain Greek yogurt topped with ½ cup blueberries

Lunch

Mexican Chopped Salad (page 165)

Midafternoon Snack

Chocolate Mint Parfait (page 231), served with 4 strawberries

Dinner

Indian Spiced Chicken and Rice (page 202)

Evening Snack

Gingersnap Oatmeal (page 236) with ½ cup nonfat milk

Per day: 1,260 calories, 97 g protein, 183 g carbohydrates, 22 g total fat, 10 g saturated fat, 27 g fiber, 2,410 mg sodium

Day 3

Breakfast

Honey Mustard BLT Sandwich (page 151)

Snack

½ medium red grapefruit

1½ ounces fat-free hard cheese

Lunch

Shepherd's Salad (page 167)

Midafternoon Snack

Apple Cinnamon Yogurt (page 232)

Dinner

Pork Lettuce Wrap (page 197), served with your choice of 1 grain

Evening Snack

Parmesan Popcorn (page 236) with ½ cup nonfat milk

Per day: 1,240 calories, 92 g protein, 181 g carbohydrates, 21 g total fat, 4 g saturated fat, 31 g fiber, 2,580 mg sodium

My Belly Melt

"I couldn't wear these pants just 5 weeks ago!"

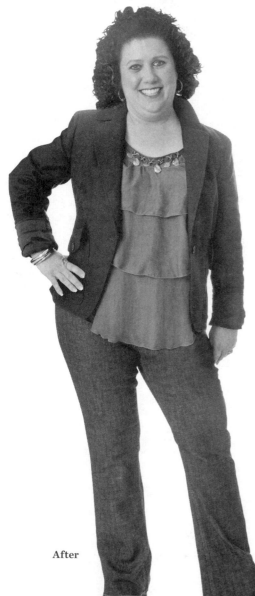

After

Andrea Miller

AGE: 40

POUNDS LOST: 19 in 35 days

POUNDS LOST IN 3-DAY RESET: 8

ALLOVER INCHES LOST: 10.5

INCHES FROM WAIST LOST: 2.5

BODY FAT LOST: 3.6 percent

Andrea Miller hardly recognizes herself. "I used to lie on the bed and cry when I tried to zip my pants," she says. Now 19 pounds lighter, she's sliding into slacks she couldn't get over her hips just 5 weeks ago. "I feel as good as I did when I was pregnant with my daughter—the healthiest time of my life."

The 3-day Reset worked magic on Andrea—she lost 8 pounds in just 3 days. That dramatic kickstart convinced her that this diet was different and fueled her

Success Story

motivation to keep going. "I tried diets before, but I never stuck with one. This program has taught me so much. I'm not hungry anymore. It's almost like I brainwashed my system." Her sleep improved, the workouts increased her energy, and everything fell into place.

Andrea's weight gain was triggered by a hysterectomy. In 6 months, she packed on more than 30 pounds. As her weight rose, her spirits plummeted. "I was so down in the dumps," she says, adding that the BMD plan was an easy education in healthy eating. "Before this program, I was a terrible eater," Andrea says. "I'd get up in the middle of the night and snack."

Getting her sleep right made a tremendous difference, she says. "My mother lives with us. At night, I always have an ear open for her and my kids, so it was

Before

hard to stay asleep." She discovered that the sugary, caffeinated sodas she drank at lunch and dinner were part of the problem. She cut them out, substituting water instead, and began practicing sleep hygiene, relaxing to get her body and mind ready for bed. The results were amazing, she says. "Not once did I get up in the night for a snack, and when I did wake up, I didn't want to eat."

Her new exercise program was a big hit with her Doberman. "Hoyt liked our morning walks, and I liked them, too." They put her in a better mood and boosted her energy. "Before, I was so tired I wanted to sleep all the time. Now I'm on a schedule, and it really works."

Andrea warded off cravings by rewarding herself along the way. When she'd lost 10 pounds, she and her son went out to eat. "I got chicken instead of a burger, but I did have a few fries." Another day she had ice cream. But each time she got right back on the program.

"I shocked myself," she says.

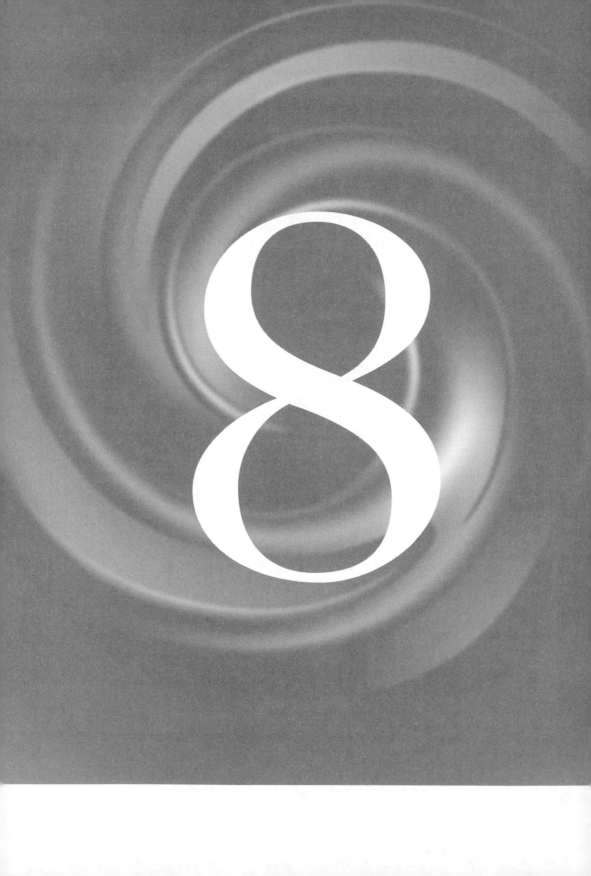

Lose Up to 19 Pounds Total in 5 Weeks

This is the phase our test panelists loved—they saw the weight falling off but said they had plenty of food and never felt hungry. The second phase runs for as long as you need to lose the weight you want. You'll be eating more calories, and your food clock will become better synchronized. At this point, even if your weight loss slows a little from the Reset phase, you'll realize that you're not hungry between meals, and many of your cravings will disappear.

When you look at the daily guidelines in the Reshape phase, you'll notice you get 300 more calories and an additional serving of grains. After reaching their target weight, some women will plateau and be able to continue using these nutrition guidelines to maintain their new firmer figure into the future. You may find you need to add an additional 300 calories in the form of a third snack or a larger breakfast, lunch, or dinner in order to maintain. The best part about this plan, however, is that you can always go back to the original Reshape or Reset dietary recommendations if you notice the numbers on the scale tipping upward.

Once you are maintaining your weight loss, the most important thing to remember is that timing is key. Continue to keep your hunger hormones in check by eating your meals close to the same time each day and by continuing to eat healthful whole foods that satisfy all your nutrition needs—especially our Sleep and Sleek foods that will keep your belly fat at bay and help regulate your many cycles.

Daily Guidelines

(See "Serving Size Guidelines" on page 118.)

- Approximately 1,500 total calories
- 5 servings grains (preferably whole grain, fiber-rich)
- 2–3 servings vegetables (3 cups total)
- 1–2 servings fruits (1½ cups total)
- 3 servings fat-free or low-fat dairy (3 cups total)
- 5 servings protein (lean meat, poultry, and fish)
- 1–2 servings fats and oils
- Maximum sodium allowance: 2,300 milligrams

Meal-by-Meal Guidelines

You don't have to follow these guidelines to a T to lose weight, but this breakdown has been shown to best keep hunger hormones in check.

Breakfast: 2 proteins, 1 grain, ½ dairy, ½ fat

Snack: ½ dairy, 1 fruit

Lunch: 1 protein, 2 vegetables, 1 grain, ½ fat

Snack: 1 dairy

Dinner: 2 proteins, 2 grains, 1 vegetable, 1 fat

Snack: ½ fruit, 1 dairy, 1 grain

Beverages: Drink two 8-ounce glasses of water before each meal and one before each snack.

Reshape 2-Week Meal Plans

(*Note:* Most meals adhere to the meal-by-meal guidelines above, although a few take a serving from one meal or snack and add it to another. You'll see these marked throughout.)

Day 1

Breakfast

Oatmeal Pancakes with Yogurt (page 152)

(uses 1 extra grain)

Midmorning Snack

1 cup nonfat cottage cheese with 1 cup sliced strawberries

Lunch

1 serving Red Lentil Soup (page 175), with 1 cup dark leafy greens drizzled with 1 tablespoon balsamic vinegar

(omits 1 grain and 1 vegetable)

Midafternoon Snack

1 cup 0% vanilla Greek yogurt

Dinner

Shrimp Scampi with Angel Hair Pasta (page 214)

Evening Snack

Lemon Almond Cheesecake Parfait (page 237)

Per day: 1,580 calories, 127 g protein, 209 g carbohydrates, 30 g total fat, 8 g saturated fat, 28 g fiber, 2,380 mg sodium

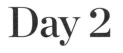

Day 2

Breakfast

2 eggs, 1 slice whole wheat bread, ½ teaspoon unsalted butter,
½ cup fat-free milk

Midmorning Snack

2 reduced-fat mozzarella string cheese sticks

1 cup frozen grapes

Lunch

White Pizza (page 181)

(uses 1 extra dairy and omits 1 protein)

Midafternoon Snack

24 raw pistachios

(uses 1 extra protein and omits 1 dairy)

Dinner

Vietnamese Noodle Soup (page 189)

Evening Snack

1 serving Chocolate Pudding (page 237) with ½ cup raspberries and
3 vanilla wafers

Per day: 1,550 calories, 91 g protein, 176 g carbohydrates, 59 g
total fat, 25 g saturated fat, 22 g fiber, 2,600 mg sodium

Day 3

Breakfast

Double-Crunch Peanut Butter and Jelly Muffin (page 153) with ½ teaspoon butter and ½ cup fat-free milk

---

Midmorning Snack

1 cup fat-free cottage cheese

1 orange

(omits ½ dairy)

Lunch

Middle Eastern Portobello Mushroom Burger (page 182)

Midafternoon Snack

Watermelon Frappé (page 232)

(uses ½ extra fruit)

Dinner

Nachos Grande (page 188)

(uses ½ extra dairy)

Evening Snack

Chai Sugar Pita Chips (page 238) with ½ cup fat-free vanilla frozen yogurt

(omits ½ fruit)

Per day: 1,570 calories, 90 g protein, 221 g carbohydrates, 45 g total fat, 10 g saturated fat, 27 g fiber, 2,470 mg sodium

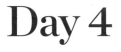

Day 4

Breakfast

1 Cinnamon Apple Muffin (page 154), served with 1 egg, scrambled with
3 tablespoons part-skim shredded mozzarella and cooked in
½ teaspoon butter

Midmorning Snack

1 small apple

¾ ounce fat-free hard cheese

Lunch

Couscous and Vegetable Salad (page 168)

(uses 1 extra dairy)

Midafternoon Snack

2 tablespoons hummus

1 cup cucumber slices

(uses 1 extra protein and omits 1 dairy)

Dinner

Orange Pork with Wild Rice and Butternut Squash (page 198), served with
½ grain of your choice

Evening Snack

Toasted Coconut and Banana Crepe (page 238)

Per day: 1,540 calories, 86 g protein, 185 g carbohydrates, 55 g
total fat, 20 g saturated fat, 21 g fiber, 2,420 mg sodium

Day 5

Breakfast

Mediterranean Pita (page 155)

Midmorning Snack

1 cup nonfat cottage cheese combined with ½ cup crushed pineapple packed in juice and sprinkled with ½ teaspoon ground flaxseed

Lunch

Southwest Tortilla Bowl (page 183)

Midafternoon Snack

Orange-Scented Ricotta with Chocolate Crunchies (page 233)

Dinner

Pasta Puttanesca with Halibut and Spinach (page 215)

Evening Snack

Strawberry Cream-Cheese Sandwich (page 239) with 1 cup fat-free milk

Per day: 1,580 calories, 118 g protein, 202 g carbohydrates, 39 g total fat, 8 g saturated fat, 29 g fiber, 2,550 mg sodium

Day 6

Breakfast

Poached Eggs with Parmesan Cheese and Spinach (page 156) with
½ cup fat-free milk

Midmorning Snack

½ cup 0% vanilla Greek yogurt

1 cup cantaloupe

Lunch

White Bean Tostada (page 184)

Midafternoon Snack

Carrot Cake Smoothie (page 233)

(uses ½ extra fruit)

Dinner

Pan-Fried Noodles with Beef, Broccoli, and Mushrooms (page 190)

Evening Snack

Fig Almond Biscotti (page 240) with 1 cup fat-free milk

(omits ½ fruit)

Per day: 1,580 calories, 113 g protein, 211 g carbohydrates, 37 g
total fat, 10 g saturated fat, 28 g fiber, 2,410 mg sodium

Day 7

Breakfast

Caprese Burger (page 157)

Midmorning Snack

Chocolate 'n' Peanut Banana (page 228) with ½ cup fat-free milk

Lunch

Orzo and Chickpea Salad (page 169)

Midafternoon Snack

1½ ounces fat-free hard cheese

Dinner

Wild Mushroom and Onion Barley with Chicken (page 203)

Evening Snack

1¼ cups puffed wheat cereal and ½ cup blueberries, with 1 cup fat-free milk

Per day: 1,530 calories, 86 g protein, 241 g carbohydrates, 36 g total fat, 8 g saturated fat, 40 g fiber, 2,330 mg sodium

Day 8

Breakfast
Huevos Rancheros (page 158)

Midmorning Snack
Fresh Fruit with Lime Yogurt Dip (page 228)

Lunch
Asian Spinach Salad with Tofu (page 170)

Midafternoon Snack
1½ ounces fat-free hard cheese

Dinner
Creamy Polenta with Shrimp (page 216), served with ½ grain of your choice

Evening Snack
S'mores (page 241), with 4 strawberries and 1 cup fat-free milk

Per day: 1,500 calories, 92 g protein, 220 g carbohydrates, 34 g total fat, 11 g saturated fat, 35 g fiber, 2,750 mg sodium

Day 9

Breakfast

Smoked Salmon Breakfast (page 159)

(omits ½ fat and ½ dairy)

Midmorning Snack

2 low-fat mozzarella cheese sticks

½ cup blueberries

(omits ½ fruit)

Lunch

Asian Pear and Mixed Baby Greens Salad (page 171), served with 1 grain of your choice

(uses ½ extra fat, ½ extra dairy, and ½ extra fruit)

Midafternoon Snack

1 cup 2% vanilla Greek yogurt

Dinner

1 serving Turkey Sausage and Chicken Jambalaya (page 212), served with 1 grain of your choice

Evening Snack

Honey-Scented Peaches 'n' Cream (page 241)

Per day: 1,560 calories, 112 g protein, 200 g carbohydrates, 42 g total fat, 12 g saturated fat, 30 g fiber, 2,530 mg sodium

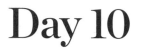

Day 10

Breakfast

Hummus Breakfast (page 160)

(omits ½ dairy)

Midmorning Snack

Café Latte (page 229) with 1 cup pineapple chunks

(uses ½ extra dairy)

Lunch

Chicken Vegetable Soup with Ginger and Lime (page 176), served with
1 grain of your choice

Midafternoon Snack

Chocolate-Malt Ricotta (page 234)

Dinner

1 serving Chicken and Couscous (page 207), served with
½ grain of your choice

Evening Snack

Mini Chocolate Chipwich (page 242), served with ½ cup fat-free milk and
½ cup berries

Per day: 1,450 calories, 85 g protein, 244 g carbohydrates, 28 g
total fat, 5 g saturated fat, 28 g fiber, 2,480 mg sodium

Day 11

Breakfast

Spicy Tex-Mex Quiche (page 161)

Midmorning Snack

1 cup fat-free cottage cheese

½ grapefruit

Lunch

Crunchy Slaw and Chicken with Peanut Dressing (page 172),
served with 1 grain of your choice

(uses ½ extra fruit and 1 extra protein)

Midafternoon Snack

2 low-fat mozzarella cheese sticks

Dinner

Fettuccine with Walnuts (page 222), served with
½ vegetable of your choice

(omits 1 protein)

Evening Snack

Raspberry Tiramisu (page 243)

Per day: 1,580 calories, 107 g protein, 181 g carbohydrates, 55 g
total fat, 11 g saturated fat, 27 g fiber, 2,140 mg sodium

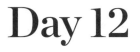

Day 12

Breakfast
Sweet Potato Hash Brown Eggs (page 162)
(uses 1 extra vegetable and omits 1 grain and ½ dairy)

Midmorning Snack
1 pear
1½ ounces fat-free hard cheese
(uses ½ extra dairy)

Lunch
Beet and Quinoa Salad (page 173)

Midafternoon Snack
Decadent Hot Chocolate (page 234)

Dinner
Pork Fried Rice (page 199)

Evening Snack
Toasted Almond and Chocolate Parfait (page 244)

Per day: 1,590 calories, 104 g protein, 186 g carbohydrates, 48 g
total fat, 10 g saturated fat, 24 g fiber, 2,460 mg sodium

Day 13

Breakfast

Breakfast Pizza (page 163)

(uses ½ extra dairy and omits 1 protein)

Midmorning Snack

1 small apple

1 tablespoon almond butter

(uses 1 extra protein and omits ½ dairy)

Lunch

Stuffed Potato Skins (page 185)

(uses 1 extra dairy and omits 1 grain and ½ fat)

Midafternoon Snack

Cheesy Lemon-Pepper Dip (page 235)

Dinner

Bulgur Lentil Pilaf with Apple (page 226)

Evening Snack

Blueberry Fluff with Ginger Crunchies (page 244)

Per day: 1,540 calories, 100 g protein, 223 g carbohydrates, 37 g total fat, 11 g saturated fat, 47 g fiber, 2,270 mg sodium

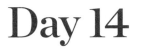

Day 14

Breakfast
French Onion Tuna Muffin (page 164)

Midmorning Snack
Baked Stuffed Apple (page 230)

Lunch
Sweet Potato and Black Bean Chili (page 177), served with 1 ounce light baked tortilla chips

Midafternoon Snack
Berry Chocolate Frozen-Yogurt Pops (page 235)

(uses ½ extra fruit)

Dinner
Chicken and Fettuccine Alfredo (page 208)

Evening Snack
Rice Pudding (page 245)

(omits ½ fruit)

Per day: 1,580 calories, 90 g protein, 258 g carbohydrates, 29 g total fat, 6 g saturated fat, 38 g fiber, 2,260 mg sodium

My Belly Melt

"I can't wait to buy some fitted T-shirts!"

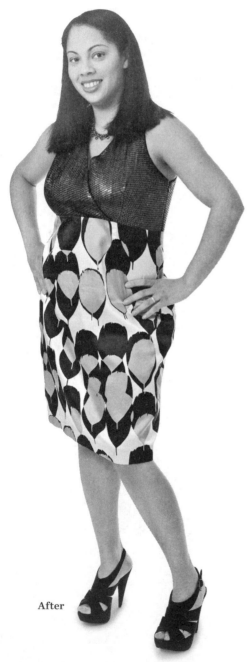

After

Idalissa Lugo

AGE: 30

POUNDS LOST: 9.2 in 35 days

POUNDS LOST IN 3-DAY RESET: 3.8

ALLOVER INCHES LOST: 3.75

INCHES FROM WAIST LOST: 1

BODY FAT LOST: 3 percent

Idalissa was battling the ultimate schedule breaker—three kids under the age of 8. "I never lost the baby weight," she says. Between juggling the schedules of her 8-year-old, 6-year-old, and 18-month-old and feeding them snacks, her weight ballooned.

But the Belly Melt Diet helped her regain control of her eating schedule as well as portion sizes, and she's thrilled at the difference in such a short time. She dropped a full size—from a 10 to an 8—in just 5 weeks, and has seen a huge improvement in how her clothes fit. "I don't need a safety pin to close the buttons on my shirt, and my belly fat is down. I can't wait to buy some fitted T-shirts!"

Idalissa lost more than 3 pounds on the 3-day Reset quick start, and seeing such great results so quickly convinced her that this program might be different from other ones she'd tried. She stuck with the meal plan—a mini-bagel and an egg for breakfast, salad with turkey for lunch, pork and brown rice for dinner—and lost 3 pounds.

After that, following the plan became easier and easier, especially with the burst of energy she got from sleeping better and exercising regularly. As for sleeping, her problem never was falling asleep, it was getting up in the morning. Until she started the BMD sleep regimen, she says, "I would drag myself out of bed." By improving her evening routine—going to bed regularly at 9:00, with a glass of water or a light snack first so she wouldn't be hungry later, and turning off the TV well before

Before

bedtime—she fell asleep faster, and began to wake up on her own. Suddenly this owl was acting like a lark.

She used a treadmill at work three times a week, and took walks with the kids whenever she could. "I don't have dumbbells, so I did the upper-body workout with a box of salt in each hand," she says. Getting regular exercise boosted her vitality and her mood.

On the food front, little changes added up to big results. She switched from whole milk to skim in her coffee, cut out sweetened soda, stuck to whole grains, and bought shopping cartsful of veggies. "I get fuller faster with healthy food. Before, I'd want seconds," she says. She knew that all the water she was drinking was helping her feel satisfied. When she got bored with the taste, she'd stir in a little Crystal Light.

Idalissa's 9-pound weight loss has whetted her appetite for more, and because she finds the program easy to follow, she's confident that she'll succeed. "I know if I keep going, I'll hit my goal. I can keep with this program because it doesn't feel restrictive. I'm never hungry."

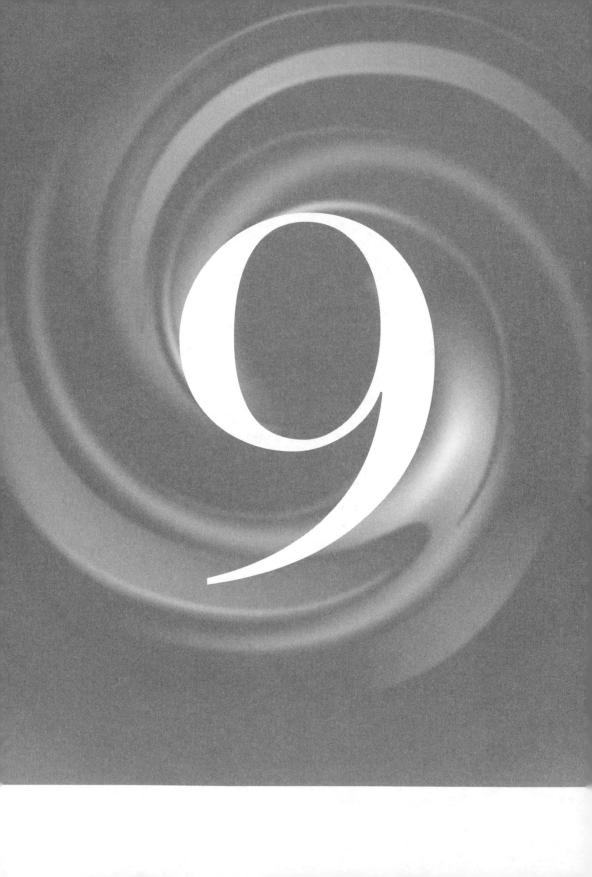

The Belly Melt Diet Recipes

These deliciously easy recipes could be found in the best cookbooks, they're *that* good. And not only will they tantalize your tastebuds, but they'll help you get off the cycle of yo-yo dieting, kick cravings to the curb, and lose the weight you want—for good!

Each recipe was specially crafted by our recipe developer and diet and nutrition expert Shari Citron, RD, to fit the Belly Melt Diet meal plan and guidelines that she created for each phase (see page 117 and page 128). And most utilize either the wonderful Sleep and Sleek foods or PMS Tamers listed in Chapter 6. Some give or take a serving from the meal-by-meal guidelines, but that's noted, so you can track that if you care to. Others can be used in either phase just by making a small adjustment. That said, if you want to pick and choose each meal, they're constructed to generally fit the meal-by-meal calorie and nutrient breakdown you need, so keeping track isn't required unless you choose to. And if you love a Phase 1 meal, feel free to make it in Phase 2. There are no restrictions in this plan at all! Bon appétit!

Recipes made with Sleep and Sleek foods

Recipes made with PMS Tamer foods

Garlic 'n' Herb Vegetable Egg Scramble

PHASE 1 • SS PMS

Prep time: 5 minutes • Total time: 15 minutes • Makes 1 serving

¼ green bell pepper, sliced

4 fresh mushrooms, sliced

¼ small onion, chopped

½ teaspoon unsalted butter

1 omega-3-enriched egg, lightly beaten

2 teaspoons chopped fresh parsley

⅛ teaspoon salt

⅛ teaspoon black pepper

1 whole wheat pita (4" diameter)

1 piece (¾ ounce) garlic-and-herb light spreadable cheese

1. Lightly coat a large nonstick skillet with cooking spray. Set over medium-high heat. Cook and stir the bell pepper, mushrooms, and onion, adding a scant amount of water if needed to prevent sticking, for 5 minutes, or until softened.

2. Add the butter and let it melt. Add the egg, parsley, salt, and black pepper. Cook and stir for 1 minute, or until the egg is set.

3. Cut the pita in half and open to form a pocket. Spread the cheese inside and fill with the egg mixture.

Per serving: 230 calories, 14 g protein, 22 g carbohydrates, 9 g total fat, 4 g saturated fat, 4 g fiber, 800 mg sodium

*uses extra ½ dairy

Breakfast

Savory Apricot-Stuffed French Toast with Tomatoes

PHASE 1 • **PMS**

Prep time: 5 minutes • Total time: 15 minutes • Makes 1 serving

1 tablespoon goat cheese, at room temperature

2 teaspoons apricot jam

2 slices light whole wheat bread

¼ cup liquid egg substitute

1 tablespoon snipped fresh chives

½ teaspoon unsalted butter

½ cup grape tomatoes, halved

⅛ teaspoon herbes de Provence

⅛ teaspoon salt

⅛ teaspoon pepper

1. Spread the cheese and jam on 1 slice of bread. Top with the remaining slice.

2. In a shallow bowl, whisk together the egg substitute and chives.

3. Coat a large nonstick skillet with cooking spray. Add the butter and heat over medium-high heat. Dip the sandwich into the egg mixture, allowing excess to run off. Cook, turning once, for 10 minutes, or until golden brown. Remove to a plate.

4. Coat the skillet with cooking spray. Set over medium-high heat. Stir and cook the tomatoes, herbes de Provence, salt, and pepper for about 2 minutes, or until just softened. Serve with the French toast.

Per serving: 230 calories, 14 g protein, 30 g carbohydrates, 8 g total fat, 5 g saturated fat, 8 g fiber, 680 mg sodium

Honey Mustard BLT Sandwich

PHASE 1 • **SS** **PMS**

Prep time: 5 minutes • Total time: 10 minutes • Makes 1 serving

3 slices extra-lean turkey bacon

1 tablespoon fat-free mayonnaise

1 teaspoon honey mustard

2 slices light whole wheat bread, toasted

½ cup baby spinach

2 slices tomato

1. Cook the bacon according to package directions.

2. In a small bowl, stir together the mayonnaise and mustard. Spread over 1 side of a bread slice. Top with the spinach, bacon, tomato, and the remaining bread slice.

Per serving: 180 calories, 14 g protein, 26 g carbohydrates, 3 g total fat, 0 g saturated fat, 8 g fiber, 790 mg sodium

Breakfast

Oatmeal Pancakes with Yogurt

PHASE 2 • **SS** **PMS**

Prep time: 5 minutes • Total time: 15 minutes • Makes 1 serving

½ cup quick-cooking oats

½ cup 0% vanilla Greek yogurt, divided

2 omega-3-enriched eggs

¼ teaspoon vanilla extract

⅛ teaspoon ground cinnamon

½ teaspoon unsalted butter

1. In a mini food processor or a blender, combine the oats, ¼ cup yogurt, eggs, vanilla, and cinnamon. Process or blend for 1 minute, or until smooth.

2. Coat a nonstick skillet with cooking spray. Add the butter and heat over medium heat. Ladle the batter in ¼ cup portions onto the pan. Cook, turning once, for 2 to 3 minutes, or until lightly browned on both sides. Serve with the remaining ¼ cup yogurt.

Per serving: 400 calories, 30 g protein, 37 g carbohydrates, 14 g total fat, 5 g saturated fat, 4 g fiber, 190 mg sodium

*uses extra 1 grain

Breakfast

Double-Crunch Peanut Butter and Jelly Muffin

PHASE 2 • **PMS**

Prep time: 5 minutes • Total time: 5 minutes • Makes 1 serving

1 light multigrain English muffin

2 tablespoons crunchy peanut butter

2 teaspoons jelly, any flavor

2 teaspoons chopped unsalted peanuts

Toast the muffin. Spread with the peanut butter and jelly. Sprinkle with the nuts.

Per serving: 390 calories, 15 g protein, 44 g carbohydrates, 21 g total fat, 3 g saturated fat, 7 g fiber, 430 mg sodium

*serve with ½ fat and ½ dairy for a complete Phase 2 breakfast

Breakfast

Cinnamon Apple Muffins

PHASE 1 OR 2 • **SS** **PMS**

Prep time: 10 minutes • Total time: 35 minutes plus cooling time• Makes 12

1 cup high-fiber cereal, crushed
⅔ cup fat-free milk
1¼ cups unbleached or all-purpose flour
¼ cup ground flaxseed
1 tablespoon baking powder
2 teaspoons ground cinnamon

½ teaspoon salt
½ cup packed light brown sugar
½ cup liquid egg substitute
1 tablespoon canola oil
1 teaspoon vanilla extract
1 cup chopped apple
¾ cup shredded carrot

1. Preheat the oven to 375°F. Place paper liners in a 12-cup muffin pan. Coat the bottoms with cooking spray.

2. In a large bowl, stir together the cereal and milk. Let stand for 5 minutes, or until the cereal is softened. In a bowl, stir together the flour, flaxseed, baking powder, cinnamon, and salt.

3. When the cereal is softened, stir in the sugar, egg substitute, oil, and vanilla until the sugar dissolves. Fold in the dry ingredients. Stir in the apple and carrot. Divide evenly among the muffin cups.

4. Bake for 22 to 25 minutes, or until a toothpick inserted in the center comes out clean. Cool in the pan on a rack for 5 minutes. Remove to the rack and cool for about 10 minutes. Serve warm if desired.

Per muffin: 130 calories, 4 g protein, 26 g carbohydrates, 3 g total fat, 0 g saturated fat, 3 g fiber, 240 mg sodium

*serve with 1 protein, ½ vegetable, and ½ fat for a complete Phase 1 breakfast
**serve with 2 proteins, ½ dairy, and ½ fat for a complete Phase 2 breakfast

Breakfast

Mediterranean Pita

PHASE 1 OR 2 • SS PMS

Prep time: 5 minutes • Total time: 10 minutes • Makes 1 serving

½ teaspoon unsalted butter
1 cup baby spinach
1 omega-3-enriched egg
2 egg whites

3 tablespoons fat-free feta cheese
½ teaspoon chopped fresh dill
1 whole wheat pita (4" diameter)

1. Coat a large nonstick skillet with cooking spray. Add the butter and heat over medium-high heat. Cook the spinach for 1 minute, or until just wilted. Remove to a plate.

2. In a bowl, whisk together the egg, egg whites, cheese, and dill. Coat the skillet with cooking spray. Set over medium-high heat. Cook and stir the egg mixture for 1 minute, or until set. Cut the pita in half and open to form a pocket. Fill with the eggs and spinach.

Per serving: 260 calories, 27 g protein, 21 g carbohydrates, 7 g total fat, 3 g saturated fat, 3 g fiber, 370 mg sodium

*serve without egg whites for Phase 1 breakfast

Breakfast

Poached Eggs with Parmesan Cheese and Spinach

PHASE 1 OR 2 • **SS** **PMS**

Prep time: 5 minutes • Total time: 15 minutes • Makes 1 serving

2 cups baby spinach

½ teaspoon unsalted butter, at room
temperature

2 slices light whole wheat bread

2 teaspoons grated Parmesan cheese

2 omega-3-enriched eggs

2 teaspoons pesto

⅛ teaspoon pepper

1. Coat a large nonstick skillet with cooking spray. Cook the spinach, adding a scant amount of water if needed to prevent sticking, for 1 to 2 minutes, or until wilted. Remove to a plate.

2. Spread the butter over 1 side of each bread slice. Sprinkle with the cheese. Place the bread in a toaster oven. Toast for 1 to 2 minutes, or until golden brown.

3. Fill the skillet with enough water to measure 1¼". Cover and bring almost to a boil over medium heat. One at a time, add the eggs to the water. Reduce the heat to medium-low, or just until the water simmers. Cook for 3 minutes, or until the egg whites are just set and the yolks are still runny.

4. Divide the toast between two plates. Divide the spinach over the toast. Using a slotted spoon, transfer 1 egg, well drained, to each slice of bread. Drizzle with the pesto and sprinkle with the pepper.

Per serving: 320 calories, 20 g protein, 21 g carbohydrates, 18 g total fat, 7 g saturated fat, 5 g fiber, 650 mg sodium

*serve with only one egg for Phase 1

**serve with ½ dairy for a complete Phase 2 breakfast

Caprese Burger

PHASE 2 • SS PMS

Prep time: 5 minutes • Total time: 10 minutes • Makes 1 serving

1 vegetable burger (2.75 ounces)
½ teaspoon canola oil
1 light multigrain English muffin

2 slices tomato
1 slice (1 ounce) fresh mozzarella
4 fresh basil leaves

1. Prepare the vegetable burger according to package directions using the oil.

2. Toast the muffin. Place the burger on the muffin bottom. Top with the tomato, cheese, basil, and muffin top.

Per serving: 320 calories, 15 g protein, 41 g carbohydrates, 15 g total fat, 5 g saturated fat, 14 g fiber, 420 mg sodium

Breakfast

Huevos Rancheros

Prep time: 5 minutes • Total time: 15 minutes • Makes 1 serving

½ tomato, chopped

¼ cup frozen corn kernels, thawed

¼ cup 50%-less-salt black beans

½ small jalapeño pepper, sliced (wear plastic gloves when handling)

½ teaspoon canola oil

1 low-carb, 95% fat-free multigrain tortilla (8" diameter)

3 tablespoons shredded reduced-fat Cheddar cheese

1 omega-3-enriched egg

⅛ teaspoon black pepper

1 teaspoon chopped fresh cilantro

1. Preheat the oven to 425°F. Coat a baking sheet with cooking spray.

2. In a small bowl, combine the tomato, corn, beans, jalapeño pepper, and oil. Place the tortilla on the baking sheet. Sprinkle with the cheese and top with the tomato mixture. With the back of a spoon, make a depression in the center of the mixture. Place the egg in the center. Sprinkle with the black pepper.

3. Bake for 8 minutes, or until the egg white is set and the yolk is still runny. Sprinkle with the cilantro.

Per serving: 300 calories, 22 g protein, 32 g carbohydrates, 14 g total fat, 5 g saturated fat, 11 g fiber, 380 mg sodium

Breakfast

Smoked Salmon Breakfast

PHASE 2 • **SS** **PMS**

Prep time: 5 minutes • Total time: 5 minutes • Makes 1 serving

1 light multigrain English muffin

2 tablespoons fat-free cream cheese

1½ ounces smoked salmon

2 thin slices red onion

½ teaspoon capers

½ teaspoon chopped fresh dill

Toast the muffin. Spread the cream cheese over the bottom. Top with the salmon, onion, capers, dill, and muffin top.

Per serving: 190 calories, 18 g protein, 30 g carbohydrates, 3 g total fat, 1 g saturated fat, 9 g fiber, 730 mg sodium

*serve with ½ fat and ½ dairy for a complete Phase 2 breakfast

Breakfast

Hummus Breakfast

PHASE 2 • **SS** **PMS**

Prep time: 5 minutes • Total time: 5 minutes • Makes 1 serving

1 whole wheat pita (4" diameter)
⅓ cup hummus
¼ small cucumber, sliced

¼ cup alfalfa sprouts
2 slices tomato
½ teaspoon flaxseed oil

Cut the pita in half and open to form a pocket. Fill with the hummus, cucumber, sprouts, and tomato. Drizzle with the oil.

Per serving: 250 calories, 11 g protein, 30 g carbohydrates, 11 g total fat, 2 g saturated fat, 8 g fiber, 470 mg sodium

*serve with ½ dairy for a complete Phase 2 breakfast

Breakfast

Spicy Tex-Mex Quiche

PHASE 2 • **SS** **PMS**

Prep time: 5 minutes • Total time: 40 minutes • Makes 4 servings

4 low-carb, 95% fat-free multigrain tortillas (8" diameter)
1 tablespoon canola oil
1½ ounces spicy jalapeño pepper chicken sausage, chopped
½ green bell pepper, chopped
½ small onion, chopped
⅛ teaspoon chipotle chile powder
4 omega-3-enriched eggs
½ cup fat-free half-and-half
⅔ cup shredded part-skim mozzarella cheese

1. Preheat the oven to 375°F. Set 4 custard cups (10 ounces each) on a baking pan. Press the tortillas into the cups.

2. Coat a large nonstick skillet with cooking spray. Add the oil and heat over medium-high heat. Cook and stir the sausage, bell pepper, onion, and chipotle powder for 7 minutes, or until the sausage is no longer pink.

3. In a small bowl, whisk together the eggs and half-and-half.

4. Divide the sausage mixture, egg mixture, and cheese among the prepared tortilla cups.

5. Bake, covering loosely with foil halfway through cooking, for 25 to 30 minutes, or until just set.

Per serving: 250 calories, 20 g protein, 17 g carbohydrates, 14 g total fat, 4 g saturated fat, 8 g fiber, 310 mg sodium

Breakfast

Sweet Potato Hash Brown Eggs

PHASE 1 OR 2 • **SS** **PMS**

Prep time: 10 minutes • Total time: 20 minutes • Makes 1 serving

½ teaspoon canola oil
2 slices extra-lean turkey bacon, coarsely chopped
½ small sweet potato, cut into ½" pieces

½ green bell pepper, chopped
¼ small onion, chopped
1 omega-3-enriched egg

1. Coat a large nonstick skillet with cooking spray. Add the oil and heat over medium-high heat. Cook the bacon, potato, bell pepper, and onion for 8 to 10 minutes, or until the bacon is crisp and the vegetables are tender. Remove to a plate.

2. Coat the skillet with cooking spray. Over medium-high heat, cook the egg for 2 to 3 minutes, or until the white is set and the yolk is still runny. Serve over the hash.

Per serving: 280 calories, 16 g protein, 12 g carbohydrates, 19 g total fat, 5 g saturated fat, 2 g fiber, 790 mg sodium

*serve without bacon for Phase 1 breakfast

**uses extra 1 vegetable serving

***serve with 1 grain and ½ dairy for a complete Phase 2 breakfast

Breakfast

Breakfast Pizza

PHASE 2 • **PMS**

Prep time: 5 minutes • Total time: 20 minutes • Makes 1 serving

1 low-carb, 95% fat-free multigrain tortilla (8" diameter)

½ tomato, chopped

½ teaspoon olive oil

1 slice (1 ounce) low-sodium turkey breast, coarsely chopped

⅓ cup shredded part-skim mozzarella cheese

1 tablespoon torn fresh basil

1. Preheat the oven to 450°F. Coat a small baking sheet with cooking spray. Place the tortilla on the baking sheet and top with the tomato. Drizzle with the oil. Top with the turkey and cheese.

2. Bake for 10 to 12 minutes, or until the cheese is melted and beginning to brown. Sprinkle with the basil.

Per serving: 220 calories, 22 g protein, 16 g carbohydrates, 11 g total fat, 4 g saturated fat, 8 g fiber, 460 mg sodium

*uses extra ½ dairy

**serve with 1 protein for a complete Phase 2 breakfast

French Onion Tuna Muffin

PHASE 2 • **PMS**

Prep time: 5 minutes • Total time: 10 minutes • Makes 1 serving

½ can (5 ounces) water-packed tuna, drained

1 tablespoon fat-free mayonnaise

½ teaspoon fresh tarragon, chopped

¼ teaspoon Dijon mustard

1 light multigrain English muffin, toasted

1 wedge (¾ ounce) French Onion light spreadable cheese

2 slices tomato

In a small bowl, stir together the tuna, mayonnaise, tarragon, and mustard. Toast the muffin. Spread the cheese over both sides of muffin. Spoon the tuna mixture onto the muffin bottom. Top with the tomato and muffin top.

Per serving: 230 calories, 21 g protein, 31 g carbohydrates, 5 g total fat, 2 g saturated fat, 10 g fiber, 780 mg sodium

Breakfast

Mexican Chopped Salad

PHASE 1 • SS PMS

Prep time: 10 minutes • Total time: 10 minutes • Makes 1 serving

¼ cup orange juice

2 teaspoons fresh cilantro, chopped

½ teaspoon grated orange peel

½ teaspoon flaxseed oil

¼ teaspoon ground cumin

¼ teaspoon salt

¼ teaspoon pepper

5 large leaves romaine lettuce, chopped

1 tomato, chopped

¼ cup 50%-less-salt black beans

6 radishes, sliced

2 scallions, diagonally sliced

3 tablespoons fat-free feta cheese

In a large bowl, whisk together the orange juice, cilantro, orange peel, oil, cumin, salt, and pepper. Add the lettuce, tomato, beans, radishes, scallions, and cheese. Toss to coat with the dressing.

Per serving: 200 calories, 16 g protein, 29 g carbohydrates, 3 g total fat, 0 g saturated fat, 7 g fiber, 760 mg sodium

Lunch

Edamame Salad with Carrot Ginger Dressing

PHASE 1 • **PMS** **SS**

Prep time: 10 minutes • Total time: 10 minutes • Makes 1 serving

2 cups mixed leafy greens

½ cup grape tomatoes, halved

¼ small cucumber, sliced

½ cup bean sprouts

¼ cup shelled edamame

2 scallions, sliced

2 tablespoons Carrot Ginger Dressing (below)

½ teaspoon toasted sesame seeds

In a large bowl, toss together the greens, tomatoes, cucumber, bean sprouts, edamame, scallions, dressing, and sesame seeds.

Per serving: 190 calories, 10 g protein, 20 g carbohydrates, 9 g total fat, 1 g saturated fat, 8 g fiber, 115 mg sodium

Carrot Ginger Dressing

PHASE 1 OR 2 • **SS**

Prep time: 5 minutes • Total time: 10 minutes • Makes 14 servings
(28 tablespoons)

3 carrots, coarsely chopped

¼ cup fresh ginger, chopped

2 shallots, chopped

¼ cup rice wine vinegar

1 tablespoon reduced-sodium soy sauce

1 tablespoon toasted sesame oil

Salt

⅓ cup canola oil

⅓ cup water

In a food processor or a blender, combine the carrots, ginger, shallots, vinegar, soy sauce, sesame oil, and salt to taste. Process or blend, while drizzling in the canola oil and water, for 1 to 2 minutes, or until emulsified. Refrigerate in a covered container for up to 1 week.

Per serving: 60 calories, 0 g protein, 2 g carbohydrates, 6 g total fat, 0 g saturated fat, 0 g fiber, 60 mg sodium

Lunch

Shepherd's Salad

PHASE 1 • **PMS**

Prep time: 10 minutes • Total time: 10 minutes • Makes 1 serving

3 falafel balls (1 ounce each)

1 small cucumber, cut into chunks

1 tomato, cut into chunks

⅛ small red onion, chopped

1 tablespoon lemon juice

1 tablespoon fresh dill, chopped

1 teaspoon tahini

¼ teaspoon sesame seeds, toasted

¼ teaspoon cracked black pepper

⅛ teaspoon salt

1. Prepare the falafel according to package directions.

2. Meanwhile, in a large bowl, toss together the cucumber, tomato, onion, lemon juice, dill, tahini, sesame seeds, pepper, and salt. Serve with the falafel.

Per serving: 220 calories, 8 g protein, 32 g carbohydrates, 9 g total fat, 1 g saturated fat, 6 g fiber, 610 mg sodium

Lunch

Couscous and Vegetable Salad

Prep time: 15 minutes • Total time: 15 minutes • Makes 1 serving

¼ cup whole wheat couscous

1½ tablespoons cider vinegar

½ teaspoon flaxseed oil

⅛ teaspoon salt

⅛ teaspoon pepper

½ cup baby arugula

1 tomato, chopped

¼ zucchini, chopped

¼ cup crumbled blue cheese

2 tablespoons snipped fresh chives

2 tablespoons chopped walnuts, toasted

1. Prepare the couscous according to package directions. Stir with a fork and let cool to room temperature.

2. Meanwhile, in a large bowl, whisk together the vinegar, oil, salt, and pepper. Add the arugula, tomato, zucchini, cheese, chives, walnuts, and couscous. Toss to coat with the dressing.

Per serving: 400 calories, 18 g protein, 30 g carbohydrates, 24 g total fat, 9 g saturated fat, 4 g fiber, 920 mg sodium

*uses extra 1 dairy

Lunch

Orzo and Chickpea Salad

PHASE 1 OR 2 • SS PMS

Prep time: 15 minutes • Total time: 15 minutes • Makes 1 serving

¼ cup whole wheat orzo

2 tablespoons lemon juice

1 teaspoon grated lemon peel

1 clove garlic, chopped

½ teaspoon flaxseed oil

¼ teaspoon salt

¼ teaspoon cracked black pepper

½ small cucumber, cut lengthwise then sliced

1 carrot, sliced

½ tomato, chopped

½ cup canned no-salt-added chickpeas

¼ yellow or red bell pepper, cut into 1" chunks

3 tablespoons roughly torn fresh basil

1. Prepare the orzo according to package directions. Stir with a fork and let cool to room temperature.

2. In a large bowl, whisk together the lemon juice, lemon peel, garlic, oil, salt, and black pepper. Add the cucumber, carrot, tomato, chickpeas, bell pepper, basil, and orzo. Toss well.

Per serving: 310 calories, 13 g protein, 57 g carbohydrates, 4 g total fat, 0 g saturated fat, 11 g fiber, 690 mg sodium

*serve without orzo for Phase 1

Asian Spinach Salad with Tofu

PHASE 1 OR 2 • SS

Prep time: 10 minutes + 30 minutes marinating time • Total time:
40 minutes • Makes 1 serving

¼ cup orange juice

2 tablespoons rice wine vinegar

1 tablespoon reduced-sodium soy
    sauce

½ teaspoon flaxseed oil

¼ cup firm lite tofu (2 ounces), cut
    into 1" cubes

2 cups baby spinach

¾ cup crunchy wonton chips

½ cup bean sprouts

2 carrots, sliced

¼ small cucumber, sliced

3 scallions, sliced

In a large bowl, whisk together the orange juice, vinegar, soy sauce, and oil. Add the tofu. Let marinate for 30 minutes. Add the spinach, chips, sprouts, carrots, cucumber, and scallions. Toss to coat with dressing.

Per serving: 280 calories, 12 g protein, 46 g carbohydrates, 7 g total fat, 1 g saturated fat, 8 g fiber, 680 mg sodium

*serve without wonton chips for Phase 1

Lunch

Asian Pear and Mixed Baby Greens Salad

PHASE 2 • **SS** **PMS**

Prep time: 10 minutes • Total time: 15 minutes • Makes 1 serving

¼ cup balsamic vinegar

½ teaspoon packed light brown sugar

2 cups mixed baby greens

½ small Asian pear, thinly sliced

½ pint cherry tomatoes, halved

2½ tablespoons crumbled blue cheese

7 walnut halves, coarsely chopped

⅛ red onion, chopped

1 teaspoon flaxseed oil

1. In a small saucepan, bring the vinegar and sugar to a boil over medium-high heat. Boil for 1 to 2 minutes, or until reduced by half.

2. Place the greens on a plate and top with the pear, tomatoes, cheese, walnuts, and onion. Drizzle with the oil and the vinegar mixture.

Per serving: 320 calories, 10 g protein, 31 g carbohydrates, 20 g total fat, 5 g saturated fat, 8 g fiber, 360 mg sodium

*uses extra ½ fat, ½ dairy, ½ fruit

**serve with 1 grain for a complete Phase 2 lunch

Lunch

Crunchy Slaw and Chicken with Peanut Dressing

PHASE 1 OR 2 • **SS** **PMS**

Prep time: 5 minutes • Total time: 10 minutes • Makes 1 serving

2 tablespoons orange juice

2 tablespoons rice wine vinegar

2 tablespoons chopped fresh cilantro

1 tablespoon creamy peanut butter

1 tablespoon water

1 scallion, sliced

½ teaspoon flaxseed oil

½ teaspoon grated orange peel

2 cups (8 ounces) coleslaw mix

½ cup shredded cooked chicken breast (2 ounces)

¼ red bell pepper, thinly sliced

¼ mango, cut into matchsticks

In a large bowl, combine the orange juice, vinegar, cilantro, peanut butter, water, scallion, oil, and orange peel. Add the coleslaw, chicken, pepper, and mango. Toss to coat.

Per serving: 300 calories, 20 g protein, 31 g carbohydrates, 12 g total fat, 2 g saturated fat, 7 g fiber, 390 mg sodium

*uses extra ½ fruit and 1 protein

**serve with only ¼ cup chicken for Phase 1

***serve with 1 grain for a complete Phase 2 lunch

Beet and Quinoa Salad

PHASE 2 • **SS** **PMS**

Prep time: 10 minutes • Total time: 10 minutes • Makes 1 serving

¼ cup whole wheat quinoa

1 cup canned sliced beets, drained

2 tablespoons red wine vinegar

1½ teaspoons chopped fresh tarragon

1 clove garlic, minced

½ teaspoon flaxseed oil

⅛ teaspoon salt

2 cups baby arugula

2 tablespoons fat-free feta cheese

1½ tablespoons pine nuts, toasted

⅛ teaspoon cracked black pepper

1. Prepare the quinoa according to package directions. Stir with a fork and let cool to room temperature.

2. In a bowl, toss together the beets, vinegar, tarragon, garlic, oil, and salt. In another bowl, toss together the arugula, cheese, nuts, and quinoa. Spoon the arugula mixture onto a plate. Top with the beet mixture. Sprinkle on the pepper.

Per serving: 330 calories, 16 g protein, 36 g carbohydrates, 14 g total fat, 3 g saturated fat, 7 g fiber, 620 mg sodium

Lunch

Toasted Pita Salad with Sardines

PHASE 1 OR 2 • **SS** **PMS**

Prep time: 10 minutes • Total time: 10 minutes • Makes 1 serving

1 whole wheat pita (4" diameter)
2 tablespoons lemon juice
1½ teaspoons grated lemon peel
½ teaspoon fresh parsley, chopped
½ teaspoon flaxseed oil
¼ teaspoon pepper
⅛ teaspoon salt

2 cups mixed baby greens
½ can (3.75 ounces) sardines, skinned, boned, cut into 1" pieces
1 tomato, cut into 1" pieces
¼ cucumber, halved lengthwise and sliced
¼ red onion, thinly sliced

1. Toast the pita and break it into bite-size pieces.

2. In a small bowl, whisk together the lemon juice, lemon peel, parsley, oil, pepper, and salt.

3. In a medium bowl, gently toss together the greens, sardines, tomato, cucumber, onion, and pita. Drizzle with the dressing. Toss to coat.

Per serving: 290 calories, 20 g protein, 32 g carbohydrates, 10 g total fat, 2 g saturated fat, 7 g fiber, 1,030 mg sodium

*uses extra 1 protein
**serve without pita for Phase 1

Lunch

Red Lentil Soup

Prep time: 10 minutes • Total time: 50 minutes • Makes 4 servings (7 cups)

1 tablespoon canola oil
3 large carrots, chopped
3 ribs celery, chopped
1 onion, chopped
2 tablespoons chopped fresh ginger
3 cloves garlic, chopped
1 cup red lentils

1 tablespoon ground cumin
¼ teaspoon ground red pepper
2 cans (14.5 ounces each) fat-free, reduced-sodium chicken broth
1 cup water
¾ cup lemon juice
¾ cup loosely packed fresh cilantro

1. Coat a large saucepan with cooking spray. Add the oil and heat over medium-high heat. Stir in the carrots, celery, onion, ginger, and garlic. Cook, stirring occasionally, for 10 minutes, or until tender. Add the lentils, cumin, and pepper. Cook for 1 minute. Add the broth and water, and bring to a boil. Cover and reduce the heat to medium-low.

2. Cook for 30 minutes, or until the lentils are tender. Remove from the heat. Working in batches, transfer the mixture to a blender or a food processor. Blend or process for 2 minutes, or until smooth. Return the mixture to the pot. Stir in the lemon juice and cilantro. Cook over medium heat for 2 minutes, or until just heated through.

Per serving: 260 calories, 16 g protein, 41 g carbohydrates, 5 g total fat, 0 g saturated fat, 10 g fiber, 520 mg sodium

*serve with 1 vegetable for a complete Phase 1 lunch
**serve with 1 grain and 1 vegetable for a complete Phase 2 lunch

Chicken Vegetable Soup with Ginger and Lime

PHASE 2 • **SS**

Prep time: 10 minutes • Total time: 35 minutes • Makes 4 servings (6½ cups)

3 teaspoons canola oil, divided
½ pound boneless, skinless chicken breast, thinly sliced
½ teaspoon pepper, divided
2 zucchini or yellow squash (8 ounces), chopped
1 sweet potato, cut into 1" pieces
2 ribs celery with leaves, chopped
2 tablespoons chopped fresh ginger
2 cans (14.5 ounces each) fat-free, reduced-sodium chicken broth
¼ cup + 2 tablespoons lime juice
¼ teaspoon salt

1. Coat a large nonstick saucepan with cooking spray. Add 1 teaspoon oil and heat over medium-high heat. Cook the chicken, turning once, for 4 minutes, or until no longer pink and the juices run clear. Remove to a plate. Season with ¼ teaspoon pepper.

2. Heat the remaining 2 teaspoons oil in the saucepan over medium-high heat. Cook the zucchini or squash, potato, celery, and ginger, adding a scant amount of water if needed to prevent sticking, for 10 minutes, or until lightly browned. Add the broth and bring to a boil. Cover and reduce the heat to medium.

3. Cook for 15 minutes, or until the vegetables are tender. With a slotted spoon, transfer the vegetables to a blender or a food processor. Blend or process for 1 minute, or until chunky. Return the mixture to the pot. Add the chicken and cook for 5 minutes, or until heated through. Stir in the lime juice, salt, and remaining ¼ teaspoon pepper.

Per serving: 180 calories, 12 g protein, 25 g carbohydrates, 4 g total fat, 1 g saturated fat, 4 g fiber, 960 mg sodium

*serve with 1 grain for a complete Phase 2 lunch

Sweet Potato and Black Bean Chili

PHASE 1 OR 2 • **SS** **PMS**

Prep time: 10 minutes • Total time: 30 minutes • Makes 4 servings (6½ cups)

1 tablespoon canola oil
1 sweet potato, chopped
1 onion, chopped
1½ tablespoons ground chili powder
1 teaspoon ground cumin
¼ teaspoon crushed chipotle chile pepper
2 cans (14.5 ounces each) no-salt-added diced tomatoes with Italian seasoning

½ cup water
1 can (15 ounces) 50%-less-salt black beans, rinsed and drained
1 bag (6 ounces) baby spinach
2 tablespoons fresh cilantro, chopped
2 tablespoons lime juice
½ teaspoon salt

1. Coat a large nonstick saucepan with cooking spray. Add the oil and heat over medium-high heat. Cook, stirring, for 5 minutes, or until the onion is softened. Stir in the chili powder, cumin, and chipotle pepper for 30 seconds, or until fragrant. Add the tomatoes and water. Bring to a simmer. Cover and reduce the heat to medium-low.

2. Cook for 10 minutes, or until the sweet potato is tender. Stir in the beans and spinach. Cook for 4 minutes, or until the spinach wilts. Remove from the heat. Stir in the cilantro, lime juice, and salt.

Per serving: 210 calories, 8 g protein, 40 g carbohydrates, 4 g total fat, 1 g saturated fat, 12 g fiber, 670 mg sodium

*serve with 1 grain for a complete Phase 2 lunch

Lunch

Gazpacho

Prep time: 20 minutes • Total time: 20 minutes + 8 hours chilling time •
Makes 6 servings (8 cups)

2 pounds tomatoes, chopped

1 cucumber, halved lengthwise, seeded, and chopped

1 yellow bell pepper, chopped

1 jar (12 ounces) roasted red bell peppers, drained and chopped

2 cloves garlic, minced

1 bunch scallions, thinly sliced

1 tablespoon grated lime peel

2 cups no-salt-added hot-and-spicy vegetable juice

¾ cup loosely packed fresh cilantro

½ cup lime juice

1 tablespoon flaxseed oil

2 teaspoons ground cumin

¾ teaspoon salt

¼ teaspoon ground red pepper

1. In a large bowl, toss together the tomatoes, cucumber, yellow bell pepper, red bell peppers, garlic, scallions, and lime peel. Transfer 3 cups to a large bowl. Place the remaining mixture in a blender or a food processor. Add the vegetable juice, cilantro, lime juice, oil, cumin, salt, and ground red pepper. Blend or process for 1 minute, or until smooth. Stir into the mixture in the bowl.

2. Cover and refrigerate for at least 8 hours or overnight to allow the flavors to blend. Serve cold.

Per serving: 110 calories, 4 g protein, 18 g carbohydrates, 3 g total fat, 0 g saturated fat, 4 g fiber, 580 mg sodium

*serve with 1 protein for a complete Phase 1 lunch

**serve with 1 protein and 1 grain for a complete Phase 2 lunch

Thai Salmon Chowder

PHASE 1 OR 2 • **SS**

Prep time: 15 minutes • Total time: 45 minutes • Makes 4 servings (8 cups)

½ pound skinless salmon fillet, cut into 1½" chunks

3 teaspoons canola oil, divided

1 pound shiitake and/or oyster mushrooms, sliced

2 carrots, sliced

1 red bell pepper, halved crosswise and sliced

1 large potato, cut into ½" pieces

1 box (10 ounces) frozen corn kernels

1 onion, chopped

¼ cup chopped fresh ginger

3 cups fat-free, reduced-sodium chicken broth

1 can (13.5 ounces) lite coconut milk

2 tablespoons minced lemongrass

½ teaspoon Thai red curry paste

½ teaspoon salt

¼ cup chopped fresh cilantro

¼ cup lime juice

1 tablespoon grated lime peel

1. Coat a large nonstick saucepan with cooking spray. Set over medium-high heat. Cook the salmon, turning once, for 4 minutes, or until opaque. Remove to a plate.

2. Add 1½ teaspoons oil to the pan. Heat over medium-high heat. Cook the mushrooms, carrots, and bell pepper, adding a scant amount of water if needed to prevent sticking, for 5 minutes, or until tender-crisp. Remove to the plate.

3. Add the remaining 1½ teaspoons oil to the pan. Heat over medium-high heat. Cook the potato, corn, onion, and ginger, adding a scant amount of water if needed to prevent sticking, for 8 to 10 minutes, or until tender. Remove half to a food processor. Process for 1 minute, or until smooth. Pour into the pan. Stir in the broth, coconut milk, lemongrass, paste, and salt. Bring to a boil. Reduce the heat to medium-low and simmer, stirring occasionally, for 10 minutes, or until thickened.

4. Stir in the cilantro, lime juice, lime peel, the reserved salmon, and the reserved mushroom mixture.

Per serving: 360 calories, 22 g protein, 44 g carbohydrates, 12 g total fat, 4 g saturated fat, 6 g fiber, 740 mg sodium

*serve with 1 grain for a complete Phase 2 lunch

Lunch

Indian Spinach with Tofu

PHASE 1 OR 2 • SS PMS

Prep time: 25 minutes • Total time: 40 minutes • Makes 4 servings (6 cups)

1 pound mustard greens, trimmed and chopped

1 bag (10 ounces) spinach, chopped

1 tablespoon canola oil

1 teaspoon cumin seeds

1 package (12.3 ounces) lite firm tofu, cut into ¾" cubes and patted dry with paper towels

2 tablespoons chopped fresh ginger

2 cloves garlic, minced

1 onion, chopped

1 jalapeño pepper, minced (wear plastic gloves when handling)

2 tomatoes, chopped

2 teaspoons curry powder

1 teaspoon salt

¼ teaspoon ground red pepper

¼ teaspoon ground cinnamon

2 teaspoons cornmeal

1. Bring a large pot of water to a boil over high heat. Cook the mustard greens for 5 minutes. Add the spinach and cook for 2 minutes, or until the greens are tender. Drain and reserve 1 cup cooking liquid. Place 2 cups greens mixture in a food processor. Process for 90 seconds, or until smooth.

2. Meanwhile, coat a large nonstick skillet with cooking spray. Heat the oil over medium-high heat. Cook the cumin seeds for 30 seconds, or until toasted. Add the tofu and cook, turning occasionally, for 5 minutes, or until lightly browned. Remove to a plate.

3. Coat the pan with cooking spray. Cook the ginger and garlic, stirring, for 1 minute, or until fragrant. Add the onion and jalapeño pepper. Cook, stirring occasionally and adding a scant amount of water if needed to prevent sticking, for 7 minutes, or until the onion is tender.

4. Stir in the tomatoes, curry powder, salt, red pepper, and cinnamon. Cook for 4 minutes, or until the tomatoes soften. Stir in the cornmeal, greens, greens puree, tofu, and ½ cup cooking liquid. Cover and cook over medium heat for 7 minutes, or until the vegetables are tender and the mixture thickens. If the mixture appears too dry, stir in the remaining ½ cup cooking liquid. Cook for 3 minutes, or until heated through.

Per serving: 140 calories, 12 g protein, 14 g carbohydrates, 6 g total fat, 1 g saturated fat, 6 g fiber, 690 mg sodium

*serve with 1 grain for a complete Phase 2 lunch

White Pizza

Prep time: 5 minutes • Total time: 30 minutes • Makes 1 serving

1 low-carb, 95% fat-free multigrain tortilla (8" diameter)

3 tablespoons goat cheese, at room temperature

½ teaspoon canola oil, divided

1 small onion, thinly sliced

¼ teaspoon sugar

1 zucchini or yellow squash (7 ounces), sliced ¼" thick

¼ teaspoon dried thyme

¼ teaspoon cracked black pepper

⅛ teaspoon salt

1. Preheat the oven to 350°F. Coat a baking sheet with cooking spray. Place the tortilla on the baking sheet.

2. Bake for 4 minutes, or until crisp. Spread the cheese on the tortilla leaving ½" border. Set aside.

3. Meanwhile, coat a nonstick skillet with cooking spray. Add ¼ teaspoon oil and heat over medium-high heat. Reduce the heat to medium-low. Cook the onion and sugar, covered, stirring occasionally, for 8 minutes, or until caramelized. Remove to a plate.

4. Heat the remaining ¼ teaspoon oil in the pan over medium-high heat. Add the zucchini or squash and thyme. Cover and cook, tossing occasionally and adding a scant amount of water if needed to prevent sticking, for 5 minutes, or until tender-crisp. Stir in the onions. Spoon evenly over the reserved tortilla.

5. Bake for 5 minutes, or until the cheese melts. Season with the pepper and salt.

Per serving: 290 calories, 18 g protein, 25 g carbohydrates, 17 g total fat, 9 g saturated fat, 11 g fiber, 520 mg sodium

*uses extra 1 dairy

**serve with 1 protein for a complete Phase 2 lunch

Middle Eastern Portobello Mushroom Burger

PHASE 2 • **SS** **PMS**

Prep time: 5 minutes • Total time: 15 minutes • Makes 1 serving

1 small portobello mushroom cap
½ teaspoon canola oil
¼ teaspoon dried Italian seasoning
⅛ teaspoon salt
⅛ teaspoon pepper

1 light whole wheat hamburger bun
2 tablespoons hummus
½ cup baby spinach
2 slices tomato
1 thin slice red onion

1. Coat a grill pan with cooking spray. Preheat over medium-high heat.

2. Place the mushroom cap on a small plate. Drizzle with the oil and sprinkle with the Italian seasoning, salt, and pepper. Grill for 5 minutes, or until soft and tender.

3. Grill the bun, cut sides down, for 30 seconds, or until toasted. Divide the hummus between each bun half. Top the bun bottom with the spinach, tomato, onion, mushroom, and bun top.

Per serving: 200 calories, 9 g protein, 31 g carbohydrates, 6 g total fat, 1 g saturated fat, 7 g fiber, 630 mg sodium

Lunch

Southwest Tortilla Bowl

PHASE 2 • **PMS**

Prep time: 10 minutes • Total time: 20 minutes • Makes 1 serving

2 slices extra-lean turkey bacon

1 low-carb, 95% fat-free multigrain tortilla (8" diameter)

½ cup fresh or frozen and thawed corn kernels

¼ cup 50%-less-salt canned black beans, drained and rinsed

½ rib celery, chopped

½ small tomato, chopped

⅛ small red onion, chopped

⅛ avocado, chopped

1 tablespoon fat-free ranch dressing

⅛ teaspoon chipotle chile powder

1. Preheat the oven to 350°F. Prepare the turkey bacon according to package directions. Drain on paper towels. Cool and crumble.

2. Meanwhile, coat a 10-ounce custard cup with cooking spray. Arrange the tortilla in the cup, gathering to fit. Place on a baking sheet. Bake for 8 minutes, or until lightly toasted and holding its bowl shape. Remove and set aside.

3. In a medium bowl, stir together the corn, beans, celery, tomato, onion, avocado, dressing, chile powder, and bacon. Spoon into the tortilla bowl.

Per serving: 270 calories, 18 g protein, 44 g carbohydrates, 7 g total fat, 0 g saturated fat, 13 g fiber, 530 mg sodium

Lunch

White Bean Tostadas

PHASE 2 • **SS** **PMS**

Prep time: 15 minutes • Total time: 15 minutes • Makes 1 serving

1 whole wheat pita (4" diameter)
1/3 cup canned no-salt-added white
   beans, rinsed and drained
1 tomato, chopped, divided
1 teaspoon lemon juice
1/2 teaspoon fresh rosemary, chopped
1/8 teaspoon salt

1/8 teaspoon cracked black pepper
1/4 cucumber, chopped
2 tablespoons fat-free feta cheese
1 scallion, sliced
1/2 teaspoon flaxseed oil
1/4 teaspoon ground cumin
2 leaves romaine lettuce, sliced

1. Preheat the oven to 375°F. Slice the pita in half through the middle to make 2 rounds. Place on a baking sheet. Coat both sides with cooking spray. Bake, turning once, for 10 minutes, or until crisp.

2. Meanwhile, in a medium bowl, mash together the beans, half of the tomato, lemon juice, rosemary, salt, and pepper.

3. In a medium bowl, toss together the cucumber, cheese, scallion, oil, cumin, and the remaining tomato.

4. Spread the bean mixture over the pita rounds. Top with the cucumber mixture and lettuce.

Per serving: 240 calories, 16 g protein, 37 g carbohydrates, 4 g total fat, 0 g saturated fat, 9 g fiber, 480 mg sodium

Stuffed Potato Skins

Prep time: 5 minutes • Total time: 45 minutes • Makes 1 serving

1 russet potato

¼ teaspoon pepper

2 slices extra-lean turkey bacon, chopped

1 cup frozen chopped broccoli, thawed and patted dry

⅓ cup shredded reduced-fat Cheddar cheese

2 tablespoons fat-free sour cream

1 scallion, thinly sliced

1. Preheat the oven to 450°F.

2. Pierce the potato all over with a fork. Wrap in a paper towel. Microwave on high power for 5 minutes, or until cooked through. Remove and allow to cool slightly. Slice the potato in half lengthwise. Scoop out all but ⅛" of the flesh next to the skin. Reserve the potato flesh.

3. Coat the potato shell with cooking spray and sprinkle with pepper. Place skin-side down on a baking sheet. Bake for 15 minutes, or until the skin is crisp.

4. Coat a nonstick skillet with cooking spray. Cook the bacon for 3 minutes, or until crisp. Crumble and set aside.

5. In a bowl, stir together the broccoli, cheese, sour cream, scallion, bacon, and the reserved potato flesh. Divide between the potato skins.

6. Bake for 10 minutes, or until the cheese is melted.

Per serving: 430 calories, 26 g protein, 62 g carbohydrates, 10 g total fat, 5 g saturated fat, 10 g fiber, 660 mg sodium

*uses extra 1 dairy
**serve with 1 grain and ½ fat for a complete Phase 2 lunch

Greek-Style Quesadilla

PHASE 2 • **SS** **PMS**

Prep time: 5 minutes • Total time: 15 minutes • Makes 1 serving

¼ cup shredded part-skim mozzarella cheese

2 tablespoons fat-free feta cheese

3 scallions, sliced

¼ cup chopped cooked chicken breast

¼ small cucumber, cubed

¼ cup grape tomatoes, halved

2 tablespoons pitted kalamata olive halves, chopped

1 tablespoon chopped fresh dill

1 low-carb, 95% fat-free multigrain tortilla (8" diameter)

½ teaspoon canola oil

1. In a small bowl, stir together the mozzarella, feta, scallions, chicken, cucumber, tomatoes, olives, and dill. Sprinkle onto half of the tortilla. Fold in half and press gently.

2. Coat a large nonstick skillet with cooking spray. Add the oil and heat over medium heat. Cook the quesadilla for 2 minutes per side, gently pressing with a spatula, or until lightly browned and the cheeses are melted.

Per serving: 360 calories, 26 g protein, 25 g carbohydrates, 20 g total fat, 5 g saturated fat, 9 g fiber, 680 mg sodium

Lunch

Baked Falafel Sandwiches

PHASE 2

Prep time: 10 minutes • Total time: 40 minutes • Makes 4 servings

Falafel:

- 8 ounces shelled edamame
- ½ small onion, chopped
- ¼ cup fresh cilantro
- ¼ cup fresh parsley
- 1 tablespoon lemon juice
- 2 cloves garlic, minced
- 1 teaspoon ground cumin
- 1 teaspoon ground coriander
- ½ teaspoon salt
- ¼ teaspoon ground red pepper

Sauce:

- ¼ cup tahini
- 3 tablespoons lemon juice
- ¼ teaspoon hot red pepper sauce
- Water

Salad:

- 4 leaves romaine lettuce, sliced crosswise
- 2 tomatoes, chopped
- ½ cucumber, seeded and chopped
- 4 whole wheat pitas (4" diameter)

1. To make the falafel: Preheat the oven to 425°F. Generously coat a baking sheet with cooking spray.

2. In a food processor, combine the edamame, onion, cilantro, parsley, lemon juice, garlic, cumin, coriander, salt, and red pepper. Process for 10 seconds. Scrape the sides of the bowl. Pulse for 10 seconds, or until the mixture is almost smooth. Shape the mixture into 8 patties. Place on the baking sheet and coat well with cooking spray.

3. Bake for 18 minutes, turning halfway through cooking time and coating the patties with cooking spray, or until crisp and browned.

4. To make the sauce: In a medium bowl, stir together the tahini, lemon juice, and red pepper. Add water 1 tablespoon at a time until the mixture has the consistency of creamy salad dressing.

5. To make the salad: In a medium bowl, combine the lettuce, tomatoes, and cucumber.

6. To make the sandwiches: Cut the pitas in half and open to form pockets. Place on a baking sheet and bake for 2 minutes, or until warm. Divide the salad, falafel patties, and sauce evenly among the pita halves.

Per serving: 250 calories, 11 g protein, 29 g carbohydrates, 11 g total fat, 2 g saturated fat, 7 g fiber, 470 mg sodium

Nachos Grande

PHASE 2 • **SS** **PMS**

Prep time: 10 minutes • Total time: 25 minutes • Makes 4 servings

¾ pound extra-lean ground beef

1 tablespoon canola oil

1 large onion, chopped

2 cloves garlic, chopped

1 tablespoon ground chili powder

1 teaspoon ground cumin

1 can (14.5 ounces) no-salt-added diced tomatoes with Italian seasoning

1 cup fresh or frozen and thawed corn kernels

¼ cup chopped fresh cilantro, divided

2 tablespoons lime juice

¼ teaspoon salt

5½ ounces baked tortilla chips

¾ cup shredded reduced-fat Cheddar cheese

1. Coat a large nonstick skillet with cooking spray. Heat over medium-high heat. Cook the beef for 5 minutes, or until no longer pink. Remove to a plate.

2. Add the oil to the skillet and heat over medium-high heat. Cook the onion and garlic, stirring occasionally and adding a scant amount of water if needed to prevent sticking, for 8 minutes, or until softened. Cook and stir the chili powder and cumin for 30 seconds, or until fragrant. Stir in the tomatoes, corn, cilantro, lime juice, salt, and the reserved beef. Cook for 1 to 2 minutes, or until heated through.

3. Divide the chips among 4 plates. Top with the beef mixture and cheese.

Per serving: 440 calories, 27 g protein, 49 g carbohydrates, 16 g total fat, 5 g saturated fat, 6 g fiber, 620 mg sodium

*uses extra 1 dairy

Dinner

Vietnamese Noodle Soup

PHASE 1 OR 2 • **SS**

Prep time: 10 minutes • Total time: 35 minutes • Makes 4 servings (10 cups)

¾ pound beef flank steak, thinly
  sliced

1 tablespoon canola oil

2 carrots, cut lengthwise and
  diagonally sliced

1 onion, halved and thinly sliced

¼ cup chopped fresh ginger

4 cloves garlic, chopped

3 cans (14.5 ounces each) fat-free,
  reduced-sodium chicken broth

4 ounces Chinese rice flour noodles

¾ pound bean sprouts

1 bag (6 ounces) baby spinach

¼ cup lime juice

2 tablespoons Asian fish sauce

1 tablespoon grated lime peel

1 tablespoon rice wine vinegar

¼ cup fresh cilantro, chopped

¼ teaspoon red-pepper flakes

1. Coat a large nonstick pot with cooking spray. Heat over medium-high heat. Working in two batches, cook half the beef for 3 minutes, or until no longer pink. Remove to a plate. Repeat with the remaining beef.

2. Add the oil to the pot and heat over medium-high heat. Cook and toss the carrots, onion, ginger, and garlic for 7 minutes, or until tender. Add the broth and bring to a boil. Add the noodles and cook for 5 minutes, or until al dente. Add the sprouts, spinach, lime juice, fish sauce, lime peel, vinegar, cilantro, and pepper flakes. Cook for 1 to 2 minutes, or until heated through.

Per serving: 340 calories, 26 g protein, 41 g carbohydrates, 8 g total fat, 3 g saturated fat, 5 g fiber, 1,070 mg sodium

*substitute 3–4 tablespoons water for the oil in Phase 1

**serve with 1 grain for a complete Phase 1 and Phase 2 dinner

Pan-Fried Noodles with Beef, Broccoli, and Mushrooms

PHASE 1 OR 2 • **SS** **PMS**

Prep time: 25 minutes • Total time: 50 minutes • Makes 4 servings

8 ounces fiber-and-calcium-enriched thin spaghetti
3 teaspoons canola oil, divided
1 bunch scallions, thinly sliced
3 tablespoons chopped fresh ginger
1½ pounds broccoli, trimmed and cut into florets
1 pound shiitake mushrooms, sliced

2 tablespoons water
¾ pound beef flank steak, thinly sliced across the grain
1 cup orange juice
3 tablespoons oyster sauce
2 tablespoons reduced-sodium soy sauce
1 tablespoon cornstarch

1. Prepare the pasta according to package directions. Drain, reserving ½ cup cooking water.

2. Coat a large nonstick skillet with cooking spray. Add 1 teaspoon oil and heat over medium-high heat. Cook the pasta, pressing down with a large plate that fits inside the skillet, for 3 minutes, or until golden. Coat the top of the pasta cake with cooking spray and invert onto the plate. Add 1 teaspoon oil to the skillet and heat over medium-high heat. Cook for 2 minutes, or until golden. Slide onto the plate. Keep warm.

3. Add the remaining 1 teaspoon oil to the pan and heat over medium-high heat. Cook the scallions and ginger for 1 minute. Add the broccoli, mushrooms, and water. Cook, stirring frequently, for 5 minutes, or until the broccoli is tender-crisp. Remove to a bowl.

4. Coat the skillet with cooking spray. Working in 2 batches, cook the beef for 4 minutes, or until browned. Remove to the bowl with the broccoli mixture.

5. In a medium bowl, whisk together the orange juice, oyster sauce, soy sauce, cornstarch, and the reserved cooking water until smooth. Add to the skillet and cook, stirring frequently, for 2 minutes, or until the mixture boils. Stir in the broccoli mixture. Cook for 2 minutes, or until heated through. Spoon over the noodle cake.

Per serving: 440 calories, 31 g protein, 65 g carbohydrates, 10 g total fat, 3 g saturated fat, 9 g fiber, 660 mg sodium

*substitute 3–4 tablespoons water for the oil in Phase 1

Orange-Apricot Mojo Beef Kebabs with Roasted Vegetables

PHASE 1 OR 2 • **SS**

Prep time: 15 minutes • Total time: 25 minutes • Makes 4 servings

¼ cup apricot preserves

1 tablespoon canola oil

1 tablespoon orange juice

1 tablespoon lime juice

2 teaspoons grated orange peel

1 teaspoon ground cumin

¾ teaspoon salt

¼ teaspoon pepper

¾ pound boneless beef top sirloin steak, cut into 1" chunks

1 large lime, halved crosswise and cut into eighths

1 large red onion, cut into 16 wedges

¾ pound cherry tomatoes

2 tablespoons fresh cilantro, chopped

1. Soak eight 12" wooden skewers in water for 15 minutes.

2. Preheat the broiler. Coat the rack of a broiler pan with cooking spray. In a small bowl, stir together the preserves, oil, orange juice, lime juice, orange peel, cumin, salt, and pepper. Set aside.

3. Alternately thread the beef with lime pieces onto 4 skewers. Thread the onion onto 2 skewers. Thread the tomatoes onto the remaining 2 skewers. Coat all with cooking spray.

4. Place the onion skewers on the broiler pan. Broil, turning once, for 4 minutes, or until tender. Remove to a platter.

5. Place the beef kebabs on the broiler pan. Broil, turning once, for 3 minutes, or until browned. Remove to the platter.

6. Coat the broiler pan with cooking spray. Place the tomato skewers on the broiler pan. Broil, turning once, for 2 minutes, or until tender. Remove to the platter.

7. Brush all the kebabs with the apricot-orange sauce. Sprinkle with the cilantro.

Per serving: 220 calories, 18 g protein, 21 g carbohydrates, 7 g total fat, 2 g saturated fat, 2 g fiber, 490 mg sodium

*omit the oil and serve with 2 grains for a complete Phase 1 dinner

**serve with 2 grains for a complete Phase 2 dinner

Dinner

Blue Cheese Burgers with Smothered Onions

PHASE 2 • **PMS**

Prep time: 10 minutes • Total time: 25 minutes • Makes 4 servings

1 tablespoon unsalted butter
1 large onion, thinly sliced
¼ teaspoon salt, divided
¼ teaspoon pepper, divided
1 teaspoon sugar
¾ pound extra-lean ground beef

1 teaspoon Worcestershire sauce
1 teaspoon Dijon mustard
4 light whole wheat hamburger
  buns, lightly toasted
¼ cup crumbled blue cheese, divided

1. Coat a large nonstick skillet with cooking spray. Add the butter and heat over medium-high heat. Cook the onion, ⅛ teaspoon salt, and ⅛ teaspoon pepper, stirring, for 5 minutes, or until the onion begins to soften. Stir in the sugar. Reduce the heat to medium. Cover and cook, stirring occasionally, for 8 minutes, or until the onion is caramelized.

2. Preheat a grill or grill pan over medium heat. In a large bowl, mix together the beef, Worcestershire sauce, mustard, the remaining ⅛ teaspoon salt, and remaining ⅛ teaspoon pepper. Shape into 4 patties. Lightly coat the patties with cooking spray.

3. Grill for 6 minutes, turning once, or until a thermometer inserted in the center registers 160°F and the meat is no longer pink. Place on the bun bottoms. Divide the onion and cheese evenly among the burgers. Cover with the bun tops.

Per serving: 260 calories, 22 g protein, 23 g carbohydrates, 10 g total fat, 5 g saturated fat, 3 g fiber, 550 mg sodium

*serve with 1 vegetable for a complete Phase 2 dinner

Dinner

Meat Loaf

PHASE 1 OR 2 • **SS** **PMS**

Prep time: 10 minutes • Total time: 1 hour 20 minutes • Makes 5 servings

1 can (8 ounces) no-salt-added
   tomato sauce, divided
1 teaspoon packed light brown sugar
1 pound extra-lean ground beef
1½ cups toasted whole wheat berry
   flakes and flaxseed cereal, finely
   crushed
1 omega-3-enriched egg, lightly
   beaten

1 carrot, grated
1 apple, grated
1 onion, grated
2 tablespoons cider vinegar
1 tablespoon Worcestershire sauce
1½ teaspoons dried oregano
½ teaspoon salt
¼ teaspoon ground allspice
¼ teaspoon pepper

1. Preheat the oven to 350°F. Coat the rack of a broiler pan with cooking spray.

2. In a small bowl, stir together ¼ cup of the tomato sauce and the brown sugar.

3. In a large bowl, mix together the beef, cereal, egg, carrot, apple, onion, vinegar, Worcestershire sauce, oregano, salt, allspice, pepper, and the remaining tomato sauce. Shape the mixture into an 8" × 4½" loaf. Set on the rack in the broiler pan.

4. Bake for 45 minutes. Brush with the tomato sauce mixture. Bake for 15 minutes, or until a thermometer inserted in the center registers 160°F and the meat is no longer pink. Let stand for 10 minutes before slicing.

Per serving: 260 calories, 23 g protein, 26 g carbohydrates, 7 g total fat, 2 g saturated fat, 6 g fiber, 410 mg sodium

*serve with 2 grains and ½ vegetable for a complete Phase 1 dinner
**serve with 2 grains, 1 vegetable, and 1 fat for a complete Phase 2 dinner

Pasta Bolognese

PHASE 1 OR 2 • **SS** **PMS**

Prep time: 15 minutes • Total time: 45 minutes • Makes 4 servings

1 tablespoon canola oil
1 onion, chopped
2 carrots, chopped
2 ribs celery, chopped
10 ounces fresh mushrooms, sliced
4 cloves garlic, minced
¾ pound extra-lean ground beef
1 teaspoon dried Italian seasoning
½ cup dry white wine

1 can (28 ounces) no-salt-added crushed tomatoes
½ teaspoon salt
¼ teaspoon pepper
8 ounces fiber-and-calcium-enriched spaghetti
½ cup fat-free half-and-half
2 tablespoons grated Parmesan cheese

1. Coat a large nonstick skillet with cooking spray. Add the oil and heat over medium-high heat. Cook and stir the onion for 2 minutes. Add the carrots, celery, and mushrooms. Cook, stirring occasionally, for 5 minutes, or until softened. With a slotted spoon, remove the vegetables to a bowl.

2. Coat the skillet with cooking spray. Heat over medium-high heat. Cook and stir the garlic for 1 to 2 minutes, or until fragrant. Crumble in the ground beef and Italian seasoning. Cook, stirring occasionally, for 5 minutes, or until the meat is no longer pink.

3. Add the wine and boil for 2 minutes. Add the tomatoes, salt, pepper, and reserved vegetables. Increase the heat to high. Bring the mixture to a boil and reduce the heat to low. Cover and simmer for 15 minutes, or until thickened.

4. Prepare the pasta according to package directions. Drain the pasta and return to the pot.

5. Stir the half-and-half into the sauce. Cook for 1 minute, or until heated through. Pour over the pasta. Toss to coat. Divide among 4 plates and sprinkle with the cheese.

Per serving: 430 calories, 29 g protein, 63 g carbohydrates, 8 g total fat, 2 g saturated fat, 9 g fiber, 490 mg sodium

*substitute 3–4 tablespoons water for the oil in Phase 1

Dinner

Steak Frites

PHASE 1 OR 2 • **SS**

Prep time: 10 minutes • Total time: 30 minutes • Makes 4 servings

4 russet potatoes, cut into ¼"-thick strips

3 teaspoons canola oil, divided

¾ teaspoon salt, divided

½ teaspoon pepper, divided

4 filet mignon or beef loin select tenderloin fillets (3 ounces each)

2 shallots, chopped

2 tablespoons brandy

½ cup fat-free, reduced-sodium chicken broth

1 teaspoon Dijon mustard

½ teaspoon dried thyme

1 teaspoon chopped fresh parsley

1. Preheat the oven to 450°F. Coat 2 baking sheets with cooking spray.

2. In a large bowl, toss together the potatoes, 2 teaspoons oil, ½ teaspoon salt, and ¼ teaspoon pepper. Divide the potatoes evenly between the baking sheets. Coat the potatoes with cooking spray.

3. Bake, turning and coating with cooking spray halfway through, for 20 minutes, or until crisp and golden brown.

4. Meanwhile, coat a large nonstick skillet with cooking spray. Add ½ teaspoon oil and heat over medium-high heat. Season the fillets with the remaining ¼ teaspoon salt and remaining ¼ teaspoon pepper. Cook for 4 minutes on each side, or until a thermometer inserted in the center registers 145°F for medium-rare/160°F for medium/165°F for well-done. Remove to a platter. Cover loosely with foil to keep warm.

5. Coat the skillet with cooking spray. Heat the remaining ½ teaspoon oil over medium-high heat. Cook and stir the shallots for 2 minutes, or until tender. Add the brandy. Bring to a boil, scraping the pan to loosen any browned bits. Add the broth, mustard, and thyme. Bring to a boil. Cook for 2 minutes, or until reduced by half. Add the parsley.

6. Divide the fillets among 4 plates. Drizzle with the sauce. Divide the potatoes among the plates.

Per serving: 300 calories, 21 g protein, 37 g carbohydrates, 7 g total fat, 2 g saturated fat, 4 g fiber, 510 mg sodium

*serve with 2 grains and omit the oil for a complete Phase 1 dinner

**serve with 2 grains for a complete Phase 2 dinner

Grilled Lamb Chops with Tomatoes and Orzo

PHASE 1 OR 2 • **SS** **PMS**

Prep time: 15 minutes • Total time: 35 minutes • Makes 4 servings

4 ounces whole wheat orzo pasta (¾ cup)

¼ cup crumbled fat-free feta cheese

2 tablespoons fresh mint, chopped

2 tablespoons lemon juice

1 teaspoon grated lemon peel

1 tablespoon canola oil

3 cloves garlic, minced

1 teaspoon crushed dried rosemary

½ teaspoon salt

¼ teaspoon pepper

8 baby lamb chops (4 ounces each)

8 plum tomatoes, halved lengthwise

1. Preheat the grill.

2. Prepare the orzo according to package directions. Drain and place in a serving bowl. Toss in the cheese, mint, lemon juice, and lemon peel. Set aside.

3. Meanwhile, in a small bowl, whisk together the oil, garlic, rosemary, salt, and pepper. Rub half of the mixture over the lamb chops. Place the tomatoes in a shallow dish. Toss in the remaining garlic mixture to coat the tomatoes.

4. Grill the lamb for 4 minutes, turning once, or until a thermometer inserted in the center registers 145°F for medium-rare. Grill the tomatoes for 3 to 4 minutes per side, or until softened.

5. Divide the lamb, orzo, and tomatoes among 4 plates.

Per serving: 390 calories, 37 g protein, 29 g carbohydrates, 14 g total fat, 4 g saturated fat, 7 g fiber, 380 mg sodium

*omit oil and serve with 1 grain for a complete Phase 1 dinner

**serve with 1 grain for a complete Phase 2 dinner

Dinner

Pork Lettuce Wraps

PHASE 1 • **PMS**

Prep time: 10 minutes • Total time: 55 minutes • Makes 4 servings

1⅓ cups water
⅔ cup brown Texmati rice
¾ pound extra-lean ground pork
2 carrots, chopped
1 red bell pepper, chopped
1 bunch scallions, chopped
2 tablespoons chopped fresh ginger
2 tablespoons reduced-sodium soy sauce
2 tablespoons lime juice
1 tablespoon dry sherry
½ teaspoon grated lime peel
¼ teaspoon red-pepper flakes
¼ teaspoon salt
1 head Boston lettuce, separated into leaves

1. Bring the water to a boil over high heat in a small saucepan. Stir in the rice and reduce the heat to low. Cover and cook for 50 minutes, or until the water is absorbed and the rice is tender.

2. Meanwhile, coat a large nonstick skillet with cooking spray. Heat over medium-high heat. Cook and stir the pork for 3 to 4 minutes, or until no longer pink. Remove to a plate.

3. Coat the skillet with cooking spray. Heat over medium-high heat. Cook and stir the carrots, bell pepper, scallions, and ginger, adding a scant amount of water if needed to prevent sticking, for 4 minutes, or until tender-crisp.

4. Add the soy sauce, lime juice, sherry, lime peel, pepper flakes, salt, pork, and rice. Cook and toss for 1 minute, or until heated through. Arrange the lettuce leaves on a platter. Divide the pork mixture among the leaves and fold into bundles.

Per serving: 260 calories, 23 g protein, 33 g carbohydrates, 5 g total fat, 2 g saturated fat, 5 g fiber, 490 mg sodium

*serve with 1 grain for a complete Phase 1 dinner

Orange Pork with Wild Rice and Butternut Squash

PHASE 2 • **SS** **PMS**

Prep time: 10 minutes • Total time: 1 hour • Makes 4 servings

2 cups water

½ teaspoon + ⅛ teaspoon salt, divided

1 cup wild rice and whole grain brown rice blend

2 teaspoons cumin seeds

3 teaspoons canola oil, divided

¾ pound pork tenderloin, thinly sliced

½ teaspoon pepper, divided

⅓ small butternut squash, cut into 1" cubes

1 leek, chopped

¾ cup orange juice, divided

1 tablespoon grated orange peel

1 tablespoon fresh parsley, chopped

1. In a medium saucepan, bring the water and ¼ teaspoon salt to a boil over high heat. Stir in the rice. Reduce the heat to medium-low. Cook for 40 minutes, or until the water is absorbed and the rice is tender.

2. Meanwhile, heat a large, deep nonstick skillet over medium-high heat. Add the cumin seeds and cook for 1 to 2 minutes, or until toasted. Remove to a plate.

3. Coat the pan with cooking spray. Heat 1 teaspoon oil over medium-high heat. Season the pork with ¼ teaspoon pepper and ⅛ teaspoon salt. Working in two batches, adding 1 teaspoon oil before the second batch, cook the pork for 1 to 2 minutes, or until no longer pink. Remove to the plate.

4. Heat the remaining 1 teaspoon oil in the pan over medium-high heat. Cook the squash and leek for 4 minutes, stirring, or until lightly golden. Add ½ cup orange juice. Reduce the heat to medium. Cover and simmer for 5 minutes, or until tender.

5. Stir in the rice, pork and cumin seeds, orange peel, and the remaining ¼ cup orange juice. Cook for 2 minutes, or until heated through. Season with the remaining ¼ teaspoon salt and ¼ teaspoon pepper. Sprinkle with the parsley.

Per serving: 350 calories, 22 g protein, 53 g carbohydrates, 7 g total fat, 1 g saturated fat, 5 g fiber, 500 mg sodium

*serve with ½ grain for a complete Phase 2 dinner

Dinner

Pork Fried Rice

Prep time: 10 minutes • Total time: 1 hour 10 minutes • Makes 4 servings

2 cups water

1 cup brown rice

3 teaspoons canola oil, divided

¾ pound pork tenderloin, thinly sliced and cut into ½"-wide strips

1 onion, chopped

1 pound bok choy, coarsely chopped

2 tablespoons chopped fresh ginger

3 cloves garlic, minced

3 tablespoons reduced-sodium soy sauce

1 teaspoon toasted sesame oil

2 teaspoons sesame seeds, toasted

⅛ teaspoon red-pepper flakes

1. Bring the water to a boil in a medium saucepan over high heat. Stir in the rice. Cover and reduce the heat to medium-low. Cook for 50 minutes, or until the water is absorbed and the rice is tender. Meanwhile, working in two batches, coat a large nonstick skillet with cooking spray. Add ½ teaspoon canola oil and heat over medium-high heat. Cook half the pork for 2 to 3 minutes, or until no longer pink. Remove to a plate. Repeat with ½ teaspoon oil and the remaining pork.

2. Add ½ teaspoon canola oil to the skillet and heat over medium-high heat. Cook and stir the onion, adding a scant amount of water if needed to prevent sticking, for 5 minutes, or until softened. Stir in the bok choy, ginger, and garlic, and cook for 2 minutes, or until tender-crisp, adding water if needed to prevent sticking. Remove to the plate.

3. Coat the skillet with cooking spray and heat the remaining 1½ teaspoons canola oil over medium-high heat. Add the rice and cook for 7 minutes, or until lightly browned. Add the pork, bok choy mixture, soy sauce, and sesame oil. Cook and stir for 2 minutes, or until heated through. Sprinkle with the sesame seeds and pepper flakes.

Per serving: 350 calories, 25 g protein, 42 g carbohydrates, 9 g total fat, 2 g saturated fat, 4 g fiber, 420 mg sodium

Smoky Spanish Stuffed Peppers

PHASE 1 OR 2 • **SS** **PMS**

Prep time: 10 minutes • Total time: 1 hour 10 minutes • Makes 4 servings

⅔ cup water

⅓ cup bulgur wheat

2 cans (8 ounces each) no-salt-added tomato sauce, divided

2 large green bell peppers, halved lengthwise

¾ pound lean ground pork

1 tablespoon canola oil

1 carrot, chopped

1 onion, minced

3 cloves garlic, minced

1 teaspoon ground cumin

1 teaspoon dried oregano

1 teaspoon smoked Spanish paprika

½ teaspoon salt

¼ teaspoon black pepper

¼ cup lemon juice

½ cup golden raisins

1. In a small saucepan, bring the water to a boil over high heat. Stir in the bulgur, reduce the heat to low, cover, and simmer for 10 to 12 minutes, or until the water is absorbed and the bulgur is tender.

2. Preheat the oven to 375°F. Coat a 13" × 9" baking dish with cooking spray. Spread 1 can tomato sauce into the dish. Arrange the bell pepper halves cut side up in the dish.

3. Coat a large nonstick skillet with cooking spray. Heat over medium-high heat. Cook the pork for 5 minutes, or until no longer pink. Remove to a plate.

4. Coat the skillet with cooking spray. Add the oil and heat over medium-high heat. Cook and stir the carrot and onion for 6 minutes, or until tender. Stir in the garlic, cumin, oregano, paprika, salt, and black pepper. Cook for 30 seconds, or until fragrant. Add the lemon juice, raisins, bulgur, pork, and the remaining 1 can tomato sauce. Bring to a simmer and cook for 2 minutes, or until heated through.

5. Divide the filling among the peppers.

6. Cover with foil and bake for 25 to 30 minutes, or until heated through.

Per serving: 330 calories, 22 g protein, 45 g carbohydrates, 7 g total fat, 2 g saturated fat, 8 g fiber, 450 mg sodium

*serve with 1 grain and substitute 3–4 tablespoons water for the oil for a complete Phase 1 dinner

**serve with 1 grain for a complete Phase 2 dinner

Mu Shu Pork

PHASE 2 • **SS** **PMS**

Prep time: 20 minutes • Total time: 45 minutes • Makes 4 servings

3 teaspoons canola oil, divided

2 omega-3-enriched eggs, lightly beaten

¾ pound pork tenderloin, thinly sliced

¼ teaspoon salt

¼ teaspoon pepper

2 tablespoons chopped fresh ginger

1 pound shiitake mushrooms, thinly sliced

1 bag (12 ounces) coleslaw mix with carrots

1 bunch scallions, thinly sliced

¼ cup rice wine vinegar

2 tablespoons reduced-sodium soy sauce

3 tablespoons hoisin sauce

8 low-carb, 95% fat-free multigrain tortillas (8" diameter)

1. Coat a large nonstick skillet with cooking spray. Add 1 teaspoon oil and heat over medium heat. Pour in the eggs and cook, without stirring, for 1 to 2 minutes, or until the bottom is lightly browned. Cover and cook for 1 minute, or until the eggs are set. Transfer to a cutting board. Roll up and slice crosswise into ¼" wide strips.

2. Season the pork with the salt and pepper. Wipe the skillet clean and coat with cooking spray. Add 1 teaspoon oil and heat over medium-high heat. Cook half the pork, turning once, for 4 to 5 minutes, or until lightly browned. Remove to a plate. Repeat with the remaining pork.

3. Add the remaining 1 teaspoon oil to the pan and heat over medium-high heat. Cook the ginger for 1 minute. Increase the heat to high. Cook and stir the mushrooms for 3 minutes, or until lightly browned. Stir in the coleslaw, scallions, vinegar, soy sauce, and pork. Cook, stirring occasionally, for 2 to 3 minutes, or until the cabbage has wilted and the pork is cooked through. Stir in the egg strips.

4. Spread the hoisin sauce on the tortillas. Divide the pork mixture among the tortillas. Roll into tubes.

Per serving: 410 calories, 41 g protein, 49 g carbohydrates, 13 g total fat, 2 g saturated fat, 21 g fiber, 660 mg sodium

Indian Spiced Chicken and Rice

Prep time: 20 minutes • Total time: 1 hour 10 minutes • Makes 4 servings

2 cups + 2 tablespoons water

2 tablespoons chopped fresh ginger, divided

¾ teaspoon salt, divided

1 cup brown basmati rice

¾ pound boneless, skinless chicken breast, cut into 1" pieces

1 onion, chopped

1 clove garlic, chopped

½ pound green beans, sliced in half crosswise

1 red bell pepper, sliced

2 teaspoons curry powder

1 cup lite coconut milk

2 tablespoons lime juice

1 tablespoon fresh cilantro

1 teaspoon grated lime peel

1. In a small saucepan, bring 2 cups water, 1 tablespoon ginger, and ¼ teaspoon salt to a boil over high heat. Stir in the rice. Reduce the heat to medium-low, cover, and cook for 45 minutes, or until the water is absorbed and the rice is tender.

2. Meanwhile, season the chicken with ¼ teaspoon salt. Coat a large nonstick skillet with cooking spray. Heat over medium-high heat. Cook the chicken, stirring occasionally, for 7 minutes, or until no longer pink and the juices run clear. Remove to a plate.

3. Coat the skillet with cooking spray and heat over medium-high heat. Cook and stir the onion, garlic, and the remaining 1 tablespoon ginger, adding a scant amount of water if needed to prevent sticking, for 5 minutes, or until softened.

4. Add the beans, bell pepper, curry powder, and 2 tablespoons water, and cook for 7 minutes, or until the vegetables are tender-crisp. Add the coconut milk, chicken, rice, and the remaining ¼ teaspoon salt. Cook for 1 minute, or until heated through. Stir in the lime juice, cilantro, and lime peel.

Per serving: 360 calories, 32 g protein, 43 g carbohydrates, 8 g total fat, 4 g saturated fat, 6 g fiber, 520 mg sodium

Dinner

Wild Mushroom and Onion Barley with Chicken

PHASE 2 • SS PMS

Prep time: 15 minutes • Total time: 50 minutes • Makes 4 servings

3 teaspoons canola oil, divided

¾ pound boneless, skinless chicken breast, thinly sliced

1 onion, chopped

1 clove garlic, chopped

1 teaspoon dried thyme

10 ounces assorted fresh mushrooms (such as cremini, button, oyster, and shiitake), coarsely chopped

2 cans (14.5 ounces each) fat-free, reduced-sodium chicken broth

2 cups whole grain quick-cooking barley

⅛ teaspoon salt

⅛ teaspoon black pepper

½ cup roasted red bell peppers, drained and chopped

1. Coat a large nonstick skillet with cooking spray. Add 1½ teaspoons oil and heat over medium-high heat. Cook and stir the chicken for 7 minutes, or until no longer pink and the juices run clear. Remove to a bowl.

2. In the same skillet, heat the remaining 1½ teaspoons oil over medium-high heat. Cook the onion, garlic, and thyme, stirring occasionally, for 2 minutes, or until softened. Cook and stir the mushrooms for 6 minutes, or until tender. Remove to the bowl.

3. Add the broth to the pan. Bring to a boil over high heat. Stir in the barley, salt, and black pepper. Reduce the heat to low. Cover and cook for 10 to 12 minutes, or until the liquid is absorbed and the barley is tender. Stir in the bell peppers and mushroom-chicken mixture. Cook for 1 minute, or until heated through.

Per serving: 380 calories, 24 g protein, 65 g carbohydrates, 7 g total fat, 1 g saturated fat, 9 g fiber, 650 mg sodium

Chicken Margherita Panini

Prep time: 5 minutes • Total time: 15 minutes • Makes 4 servings

¾ pound boneless, skinless chicken breast, thinly sliced

¼ cup light Italian salad dressing

8 slices (1½ ounces each) crusty whole grain bread

2 tablespoons sun-dried-tomato pesto

4 ounces fresh mozzarella cheese

2 tomatoes, sliced

12 fresh basil leaves

1. Coat a nonstick grill pan or a nonstick skillet with cooking spray. Heat over medium-high heat. Brush the chicken breast with salad dressing.

2. Grill the chicken for 6 minutes, turning once, or until no longer pink and the juices run clear. Remove to a platter.

3. Set the bread on a work surface. Coat the top sides of 4 slices with pesto. Divide the mozzarella, tomatoes, basil, and chicken evenly over the bread. Top with the remaining bread.

4. Place the panini on the grill pan or skillet. Cook, turning once and pressing down with a heavy pot, for 5 minutes, or until the bread is golden and the cheese is melted.

Per serving: 430 calories, 34 g protein, 41 g carbohydrates, 14 g total fat, 6 g saturated fat, 7 g fiber, 550 mg sodium

*uses extra ½ dairy

**serve with ½ vegetable for a complete Phase 2 dinner

Dinner

Chicken Kebabs with Tabbouleh

PHASE 1 OR 2 • PMS

Prep time: 15 minutes • Total time: 1 hour 15 minutes • Makes 4 servings

1 cup bulgur wheat
1 cup boiling water
1 pint grape tomatoes, halved
1 bunch scallions, finely chopped
½ cucumber, cut into ½" pieces
⅓ cup lemon juice
2 tablespoons fresh parsley, chopped
2 tablespoons fresh mint, chopped

1 tablespoon canola oil
1 teaspoon ground cumin, divided
½ teaspoon salt, divided
½ teaspoon pepper, divided
¼ teaspoon ground coriander
¾ pound boneless, skinless chicken breast, cut into 1" chunks
1 red onion, cut into eighths

1. In a large bowl, stir together the bulgur and water. Let stand for 1 hour, or until the water is absorbed and the bulgur is tender.

2. Stir in the tomatoes, scallions, cucumber, lemon juice, parsley, mint, oil, ½ teaspoon cumin, ¼ teaspoon salt, and ¼ teaspoon pepper.

3. Meanwhile, preheat the grill. In a small bowl, combine the coriander, the remaining ½ teaspoon cumin, the remaining ¼ teaspoon salt, and the remaining ¼ teaspoon pepper. Alternately thread the chicken and onion onto 4 metal skewers (12" long). Coat the kebabs with cooking spray and sprinkle with the seasoning mixture.

4. Grill for 8 to 10 minutes, or until the chicken is no longer pink and the juices run clear. Serve with the tabbouleh.

Per serving: 290 calories, 24 g protein, 38 g carbohydrates, 6 g total fat, 1 g saturated fat, 10 g fiber, 360 mg sodium

*omit oil and serve with 1 grain for a complete Phase 1 dinner
**serve with 1 grain for a complete Phase 2 dinner

Chipotle Pulled Chicken Sandwiches with Slaw

PHASE 2 • **SS** **PMS**

Prep time: 15 minutes • Total time: 30 minutes + 1 hour marinating time • Makes 4 servings

Coleslaw:
- 1 bag (12 ounces) shredded coleslaw mix
- ½ cup fat-free plain yogurt
- 1 small red onion, thinly sliced
- 2 tablespoons lime juice
- 2 tablespoons fresh cilantro, chopped
- 2 teaspoons grated lime peel
- ¼ teaspoon salt
- ⅛ teaspoon black pepper

Sandwiches:
- 1 tablespoon canola oil
- 1 onion, chopped
- ½ teaspoon crushed chipotle chile pepper
- 1 clove garlic, chopped
- ½ cup no-salt-added ketchup
- ½ cup no-salt-added tomato sauce
- 2 tablespoons orange juice
- ½ teaspoon grated orange peel
- ½ pound rotisserie chicken breast, shredded
- 4 light whole wheat hamburger buns
- 4 large leaves green lettuce

1. To make the coleslaw: In a large bowl, stir together the slaw mix, yogurt, onion, lime juice, cilantro, lime peel, salt, and black pepper. Cover and let marinate for 1 hour.

2. To make the sandwiches: Coat a large nonstick skillet with cooking spray. Add the oil and heat over medium heat. Cook the onion and chile pepper, stirring occasionally, for 7 minutes, or until tender. Stir in the garlic and cook for 1 minute. Stir in the ketchup, tomato sauce, orange juice, and orange peel. Bring to a boil. Reduce the heat to medium-low. Stir in the chicken and cook for 1 to 2 minutes, or until heated through.

3. Divide the buns among 4 plates. Divide the lettuce and chicken mixture among the buns. Serve with the coleslaw.

Per serving: 320 calories, 23 g protein, 42 g carbohydrates, 9 g total fat, 2 g saturated fat, 7 g fiber, 590 mg sodium

Chicken and Couscous

Prep time: 15 minutes • Total time: 35 minutes • Makes 4 servings

3 teaspoons canola oil, divided

¾ pound boneless, skinless chicken breast, cut into 1" pieces

2 carrots, sliced

2 ribs celery, sliced

1 cup fat-free, reduced-sodium chicken broth

1 cup orange juice

¼ teaspoon salt

¼ teaspoon black pepper

1 cup whole wheat couscous

¼ cup currants

½ cup roasted red bell peppers, drained and chopped

4 scallions, sliced

¼ cup pitted kalamata olives, chopped

1. Coat a large nonstick skillet with cooking spray. Add 1½ teaspoons oil and heat over medium-high heat. Cook the chicken, stirring occasionally, for 7 minutes, or until the chicken is no longer pink and the juices run clear. With a slotted spoon, remove the chicken to a plate.

2. Add the remaining 1½ teaspoons oil to the pan and heat over medium-high heat. Cook and stir the carrots and celery for 5 minutes, or until tender-crisp.

3. Stir in the broth, orange juice, salt, and black pepper. Bring to a boil over high heat. Stir in the couscous, currants, and chicken. Reduce the heat to low. Cover and simmer for 5 minutes, or until the liquid is absorbed and the couscous is tender. Fluff with a fork. Stir in the bell peppers, scallions, and olives.

Per serving: 410 calories, 26 g protein, 59 g carbohydrates, 9 g total fat, 2 g saturated fat, 8 g fiber, 550 mg sodium

*serve with ½ grain for a complete Phase 2 dinner

Chicken and Fettuccine Alfredo

PHASE 2 • SS PMS

Prep time: 10 minutes • Total time: 30 minutes • Makes 4 servings

8 ounces fiber-and-calcium-enriched fettuccine pasta

3 teaspoons canola oil, divided

¾ pound boneless, skinless chicken breast, thinly sliced

1 zucchini, halved lengthwise and sliced

3 cloves garlic, chopped

1 cup fat-free half-and-half

¼ cup fat-free cream cheese

¼ cup grated Parmesan cheese

¼ cup snipped chives

¼ teaspoon salt

¼ teaspoon cracked black pepper

1 tablespoon fresh parsley, chopped

1. Prepare the pasta according to package directions. Drain and reserve ¼ cup cooking water.

2. Coat a large nonstick skillet with cooking spray. Add ½ teaspoon oil and heat over medium-high heat. Working in two batches, cook half the chicken for 3 minutes, or until no longer pink and the juices run clear. Remove to a plate. Repeat with ½ teaspoon oil and the remaining chicken.

3. Heat the remaining 2 teaspoons oil in the pan over medium-high heat. Cook the zucchini and garlic, stirring occasionally and adding a scant amount of water if needed to prevent sticking, for 5 minutes, or until tender-crisp. Remove to the plate.

4. Combine the half-and-half, cream cheese, and Parmesan in the pan. Cook and whisk for 2 minutes, or until smooth. Stir in the chives, salt, pepper, and the reserved chicken, zucchini, pasta, and cooking water. Cook for 1 minute, or until heated through. Sprinkle with the parsley.

Per serving: 380 calories, 30 g protein, 50 g carbohydrates, 8 g total fat, 2 g saturated fat, 6 g fiber, 420 mg sodium

Dinner

Oven-Fried Parmesan Chicken Fingers

PHASE 1 OR 2 • SS PMS

Prep time: 5 minutes • Total time: 20 minutes • Makes 4 servings

¾ cup whole wheat panko bread
  crumbs

¼ cup grated Parmesan cheese

2 tablespoons fresh parsley, chopped

1 teaspoon garlic powder

1 omega-3-enriched egg

1 teaspoon water

¾ pound chicken tenders

¼ teaspoon salt

¼ teaspoon pepper

1. Preheat the oven to 375°F. Coat a baking sheet with cooking spray.

2. In a shallow bowl, combine the bread crumbs, cheese, parsley, and garlic powder. In another shallow bowl, whisk together the egg and water. Season the chicken with salt and pepper. One at a time, dip each tender into the egg mixture and then into the bread crumb mixture. Place the tenders on the baking sheet. Coat with cooking spray.

3. Bake for 12 to 15 minutes, turning once and coating with cooking spray, or until no longer pink and the juices run clear.

Per serving: 320 calories, 18 g protein, 24 g carbohydrates, 16 g total fat, 4 g saturated fat, 3 g fiber, 640 mg sodium

*serve with 2 grains and 1 vegetable for a complete Phase 1 dinner

**serve with 2 grains, 1 fat, and 1 vegetable for a complete Phase 2 dinner

Dinner

Chicken Pot Pie

PHASE 1 OR 2 • **SS** **PMS**

Prep time: 30 minutes • Total time: 1 hour 20 minutes • Makes 4 servings

3 teaspoons canola oil, divided

¾ pound boneless, skinless chicken breast, cut into 1" pieces

2 ribs celery, sliced

1 onion, chopped

4 small red potatoes, cut into ½" cubes

2 carrots, sliced

1 cup frozen baby peas, thawed

3 tablespoons water

1 tablespoon unbleached or all-purpose flour

1½ teaspoons dried thyme

1½ cups fat-free half-and-half

½ teaspoon salt

¼ teaspoon pepper

¼ cup ground flaxseed

2 tablespoons fresh parsley, chopped

5 sheets frozen phyllo dough, thawed

Butter-flavored cooking spray

1. Preheat the oven to 350°F. Coat an 11" × 7" baking dish with cooking spray.

2. Coat a large nonstick skillet with cooking spray. Heat 1½ teaspoons oil over medium-high heat. Cook the chicken, stirring occasionally, for 5 minutes, or until no longer pink and the juices run clear. Remove to a bowl.

3. Heat the remaining 1½ teaspoons oil over medium-high heat. Cook the celery and onion, stirring occasionally, for 3 minutes, or until softened. Add the potatoes, carrots, peas, and water. Cook for 8 minutes, stirring, or until tender. Add the flour and thyme; cook for 1 minute. Stir in the half-and-half, salt, and pepper for 2 minutes, or until the mixture boils and thickens. Stir in the chicken. Transfer to the baking dish.

4. Meanwhile, in a small bowl, combine the flaxseed and parsley. Place 1 sheet phyllo on a work surface. Spray with the cooking spray and sprinkle with one-quarter of the flaxseed mixture. Repeat layering with remaining phyllo, cooking spray, and flaxseed mixture. Place the phyllo stack on top of the filling in baking dish, folding edges up to fit. Make several small slits in the top. Coat with the cooking spray. Bake for 12 to 15 minutes, or until golden brown. Cover with foil and bake for 10 to 15 minutes, or until the filling is bubbly.

Per serving: 390 calories, 26 g protein, 45 g carbohydrates, 12 g total fat, 3 g saturated fat, 7 g fiber, 670 mg sodium

*substitute 3–4 tablespoons water for the oil and serve with 1 grain for Phase 1 dinner

**serve with 1 grain for a complete Phase 2 dinner

Dinner

Greek Lemon and Chicken Soup

PHASE 1 OR 2 • **SS** **PMS**

Prep time: 10 minutes • Total time: 30 minutes • Makes 4 servings (6 cups)

3 teaspoons canola oil, divided

¾ pound boneless, skinless chicken
breast, cut into 2" pieces

½ teaspoon pepper, divided

2 cans (14.5 ounces each) fat-free,
reduced-sodium chicken broth

½ cup instant brown rice

2 teaspoons Greek seasoning

2 omega-3-enriched eggs

½ cup lemon juice, divided

4 cups baby spinach

¼ cup fresh dill, chopped

¼ teaspoon salt

1. Coat a large nonstick saucepan with cooking spray. Add 1½ teaspoons oil and heat over medium-high heat. Season the chicken with ¼ teaspoon pepper. Working in two batches, cook half the chicken for 2 to 3 minutes, turning halfway through cooking, or until no longer pink and the juices run clear. Remove to a plate. Repeat with remaining 1½ teaspoons oil and the remaining chicken.

2. In the pan, bring the broth, rice, and Greek seasoning to a boil over high heat. Reduce the heat to medium-low. Cover and cook for 10 minutes, or until the rice is tender.

3. In a medium bowl, whisk the eggs and ¼ cup lemon juice. Whisk in 2 tablespoons hot broth from the pan. Whisking constantly, gradually pour the eggs into the hot but not boiling soup. Stir in the spinach and cook for 1 minute, or until wilted. Stir in the dill, salt, the remaining ¼ cup lemon juice, and the remaining ¼ teaspoon pepper.

Per serving: 260 calories, 24 g protein, 23 g carbohydrates, 9 g total fat, 2 g saturated fat, 2 g fiber, 710 mg sodium

*serve with 1½ grains, ½ vegetable, and omit oil for a complete Phase 1 dinner
**serve with 1½ grains and ½ vegetable for a complete Phase 2 dinner

Dinner

Turkey Sausage and Chicken Jambalaya

PHASE 2 • **SS** **PMS**

Prep time: 10 minutes • Total time: 35 minutes • Makes 4 servings

3 teaspoons canola oil, divided

6 ounces boneless, skinless chicken breast, cut into 1½" chunks

6 ounces spicy jalapeño pepper turkey sausage, cut into ¼"-thick slices

2 large carrots, chopped

2 ribs celery, chopped

1 large onion, chopped

2 cloves garlic, chopped

1 cup quick-cooking brown rice

1 can (14.5 ounces) no-salt-added diced tomatoes with Italian seasoning

½ cup water

¼ teaspoon salt

¼ teaspoon pepper

1. Coat a large, deep nonstick skillet with cooking spray. Add 1½ teaspoons oil and heat over medium-high heat. Cook and stir the chicken for 4 minutes, or until no longer pink and the juices run clear. Remove to a plate.

2. Coat the pan with cooking spray. Cook the sausage for 5 minutes, or until no longer pink. Remove to the plate.

3. Heat the remaining 1½ teaspoons oil over medium-high heat. Cook the carrots, celery, onion, and garlic, stirring occasionally, for 10 minutes, or until tender.

4. Stir in the rice, tomatoes, water, salt, pepper, the reserved chicken, and the reserved sausage. Bring to a boil. Reduce the heat to medium-low. Cover and cook for 10 minutes, or until the liquid is absorbed and the rice is tender.

Per serving: 280 calories, 18 g protein, 30 g carbohydrates, 10 g total fat, 3 g saturated fat, 4 g fiber, 540 mg sodium

*serve with 1 grain for a complete Phase 2 dinner

Toasted Quinoa with Shrimp, Grapefruit, and Vegetables

PHASE 1 • **PMS**

Prep time: 25 minutes • Total time: 45 minutes • Makes 4 servings

1 cup quinoa

1¼ cups grapefruit juice, strained

1 cup water

¼ teaspoon salt

¾ pound large shrimp, peeled and deveined

1 zucchini, quartered lengthwise and sliced

1 orange bell pepper, chopped

3 scallions, diagonally sliced

2 tablespoons minced crystallized ginger

2 teaspoons minced fresh thyme

1 tablespoon seasoned rice wine vinegar

1 large grapefruit, separated into wedges

1. In a large, heavy saucepan over medium heat, cook the quinoa for 2 to 3 minutes, or until lightly toasted and the quinoa starts to pop. Stir in the grapefruit juice, water, and salt. Increase the heat to high and bring to a boil. Reduce the heat to low. Cover and simmer for 15 minutes, or until the liquid is absorbed and the quinoa is tender.

2. Meanwhile, coat a large nonstick skillet with cooking spray over medium-high heat. Cook the shrimp for 2 minutes, stirring, or until opaque. Remove to a plate.

3. Coat the pan with cooking spray. Cook the zucchini, bell pepper, scallions, ginger, and thyme, stirring frequently, for 5 minutes, or until tender-crisp. Stir in the vinegar, shrimp, and quinoa. Divide the mixture among 4 plates. Top with the grapefruit.

Per serving: 310 calories, 23 g protein, 47 g carbohydrates, 4 g total fat, 0 g saturated fat, 6 g fiber, 850 mg sodium

*serve with ½ grain for a complete Phase 1 dinner

Dinner

Shrimp Scampi with Angel Hair Pasta

PHASE 2 • **SS**

Prep time: 20 minutes • Total time: 30 minutes • Makes 4 servings

8 ounces fiber-and-calcium-enriched angel-hair pasta

3 teaspoons canola oil, divided

1 pound asparagus, trimmed and cut into 1" lengths

1 red bell pepper, cut into thin strips

4 cloves garlic, minced

1½ teaspoons Italian seasoning

¾ pound large shrimp, peeled and deveined

1½ tablespoons cornstarch

1 cup low-fat, reduced-sodium chicken broth

¼ cup lemon juice

¼ teaspoon black pepper

⅛ teaspoon salt

2 tablespoons fresh parsley, chopped

2 teaspoons grated lemon peel

2 tablespoons grated Parmesan cheese

1. Prepare the pasta according to package directions. Drain and reserve 1 cup cooking water.

2. Meanwhile, coat a large nonstick skillet with cooking spray. Add 1½ teaspoons oil. Heat over medium-high heat. Cook the asparagus and bell pepper for 7 minutes, or until tender-crisp. Remove to a plate.

3. Heat the remaining 1½ teaspoons oil in the skillet over medium heat. Cook and stir the garlic and Italian seasoning for 1 minute. Cook and toss the shrimp for about 2 minutes, or until the shrimp are opaque.

4. Place the cornstarch in a medium bowl. Whisk in the broth, lemon juice, and pasta water until smooth. Add to the pan. Cook and stir for 1 minute, or until the sauce has thickened slightly. Stir in the vegetables, black pepper, and salt. Cook for 1 minute, or until heated through. Remove from the heat. Stir in the parsley and lemon peel.

5. Divide the pasta among 4 plates and sprinkle with the cheese.

Per serving: 340 calories, 25 g protein, 52 g carbohydrates, 6 g total fat, 1 g saturated fat, 8 g fiber, 840 mg sodium

Pasta Puttanesca with Halibut and Spinach

PHASE 2 • **SS** **PMS**

Prep time: 10 minutes • Total time: 25 minutes • Makes 4 servings

8 ounces fiber-and-calcium-
   enriched thin spaghetti
3 teaspoons canola oil, divided
¾ pound halibut fillets, cut into
   1½" pieces
¼ cup pitted kalamata olives,
   chopped
2 tablespoons capers
1 tablespoon fresh parsley, chopped

3 cloves garlic, minced
½ teaspoon red-pepper flakes
¼ teaspoon anchovy paste
1 can (14.5 ounces) no-salt-added
   diced tomatoes with Italian
   seasoning
2 cups baby spinach
1 tablespoon grated Parmesan
   cheese

1. Cook the pasta according to package directions.

2. Meanwhile, coat a large nonstick saucepan with cooking spray. Add 1 teaspoon oil and heat over medium heat. Working in two batches, cook half the halibut for 2 to 3 minutes, or until the fish flakes easily. Remove to a plate. Repeat with 1 teaspoon oil and the remaining halibut.

3. Heat the remaining 1 teaspoon oil over medium heat. Cook and stir the olives, capers, parsley, garlic, pepper flakes, and anchovy paste for 45 seconds, or until fragrant. Stir in the tomatoes. Cover and simmer for 5 minutes.

4. Stir in the spinach and cook for 1 minute, or until the spinach wilts slightly. Add the pasta and fish. Cook for 1 to 2 minutes, or until heated through. Sprinkle with the cheese.

Per serving: 440 calories, 21 g protein, 48 g carbohydrates, 20 g total fat, 4 g saturated fat, 7 g fiber, 430 mg sodium

Dinner

Creamy Polenta with Shrimp

PHASE 2 • **PMS**

Prep time: 10 minutes • Total time: 55 minutes • Makes 4 servings

½ cup dry-packed sun-dried
  tomatoes
5½ cups water, divided
1 cup corn grits
¼ cup grated Parmesan cheese
3 teaspoons unsalted butter, divided
½ teaspoon salt

½ teaspoon pepper, divided
¾ pound large shrimp, peeled and
  deveined
1 onion, chopped
4 cloves garlic, chopped
1 tablespoon dried basil
1 pound tomatoes, coarsely chopped

1. In a microwaveable bowl, combine the sun-dried tomatoes with 1½ cups water. Microwave on high power for 1 minute, or until boiling. Remove and let stand for 30 minutes, or until softened.

2. Meanwhile, bring the remaining 4 cups water to a boil in a medium saucepan over high heat. Gradually whisk in the grits. Reduce the heat to medium-low. Cook, stirring frequently, for 30 minutes, or until the mixture is very thick. Remove from the heat and stir in the cheese, 2 teaspoons butter, salt, and ¼ teaspoon pepper.

3. Drain and reserve the tomato liquid.

4. Coat a large nonstick skillet with cooking spray. Heat ½ teaspoon butter over medium-high heat. Season the shrimp with the remaining ¼ teaspoon pepper. Cook for 1 to 2 minutes, or until the shrimp are opaque. Remove to a plate.

5. Heat the remaining ½ teaspoon butter over medium heat. Cook the onion, adding scant amounts of the reserved tomato water if needed to prevent sticking, for 8 minutes, or until tender. Cook and stir the garlic, basil, and sun-dried tomatoes for 30 seconds, or until fragrant. Stir in the fresh tomatoes and the remaining sun-dried-tomato liquid. Reduce the heat to medium-low. Cover and cook for 15 minutes, or until the mixture is thickened.

6. Stir in the shrimp and cook for 1 minute, or until heated through. Divide the polenta among 4 plates. Top with the shrimp and sauce.

Per serving: 330 calories, 21 g protein, 46 g carbohydrates, 6 g total fat, 3 g saturated fat, 8 g fiber, 980 mg sodium

*serve with ½ grain for a complete Phase 2 dinner

Dinner

Pan-Seared Salmon over Kale

PHASE 1 OR 2 • **SS** **PMS**

Prep time: 10 minutes • Total time: 35 minutes • Makes 4 servings

3 teaspoons canola oil, divided

1 small onion, chopped

1 cup orange juice

1 cup quinoa

1 can (14.5 ounces) low-fat, reduced-sodium chicken broth, divided

2 tablespoons pumpkin seeds, toasted

2 tablespoons fresh cilantro, chopped

4 skinless salmon fillets (3 ounces each)

1 teaspoon cinnamon-chipotle rub

1 bag (16 ounces) chopped kale

½ teaspoon salt, divided

¼ teaspoon pepper, divided

1. Coat a medium saucepan with cooking spray. Add 1½ teaspoons oil and heat over medium-high heat. Cook the onion for 6 minutes, or until tender. Add the orange juice, quinoa, and 1 cup broth. Increase the heat to high and bring to a boil. Reduce the heat to low. Cover and simmer for 15 to 20 minutes, or until the liquid is absorbed and the quinoa is tender. Fluff with a fork. Stir in the pumpkin seeds and cilantro. Cover and set aside.

2. Season the salmon with the cinnamon-chipotle rub. Coat a large nonstick skillet with cooking spray. Add the remaining 1½ teaspoons oil and heat over medium-high heat. Cook the fillets for 7 minutes. Turning once, or until opaque. Remove to a serving platter. Cover loosely with foil to keep warm.

3. Wipe the skillet clean. Coat with cooking spray. Cook half the kale, ¼ teaspoon salt, ⅛ teaspoon pepper, and half of the remaining broth. Cover and cook, stirring occasionally, for 3 to 4 minutes, or until tender. Remove to the platter with the salmon. Repeat with the remaining kale, remaining salt, remaining pepper, and remaining broth.

4. Divide the quinoa among 4 plates. Top with the salmon and kale.

Per serving: 450 calories, 31 g protein, 48 g carbohydrates, 16 g total fat, 3 g saturated fat, 6 g fiber, 680 mg sodium

*substitute 3–4 tablespoons water for the oil for Phase 1

**serve with ½ grain for a complete Phase 2 dinner

Cajun Oven-Fried Fish and Chips

PHASE 1 OR 2 • **SS** **PMS**

Prep time: 10 minutes • Total time: 40 minutes • Makes 4 servings

4 sweet potatoes, cut into ¼"-thick rounds
1 tablespoon canola oil
1 teaspoon ground coriander
¼ teaspoon salt
¼ teaspoon pepper
¾ cup whole wheat panko bread crumbs

2 scallions, finely chopped
2 tablespoons reduced-fat mayonnaise
1½ teaspoons Cajun seasoning
4 cod fillets (3 ounces each)
½ lemon, cut into 4 wedges

1. Preheat the oven to 425°F. Coat 3 baking sheets with cooking spray.

2. In a large bowl, toss together the potatoes, oil, coriander, salt, and pepper. Evenly divide the potatoes between 2 baking sheets.

3. Bake, turning and recoating with cooking spray once, for 20 minutes, or until golden brown.

4. Meanwhile, in a shallow bowl, combine the bread crumbs and scallions. In another shallow bowl, combine the mayonnaise and Cajun seasoning. Place the cod on a work surface. Spread both sides evenly with the mayonnaise mixture. One at a time, dip the fillets into the bread crumb mixture to coat. Place on the remaining baking sheet. Coat both sides of the fillets with cooking spray.

5. Bake for 10 minutes, turning once, or until the fish flakes easily. Serve with the lemon wedges and potatoes.

Per serving: 330 calories, 19 g protein, 47 g carbohydrates, 7 g total fat, 1 g saturated fat, 8 g fiber, 720 mg sodium

*serve with 2 grains and omit oil for a complete Phase 1 dinner
**serve with 2 grains for a complete Phase 2 dinner

Crab Cakes

PHASE 2 • **SS** **PMS**

Prep time: 15 minutes • Total time: 30 minutes • Makes 4 servings

3 cans (6 ounces each) crabmeat, drained and picked through

2 omega-3-enriched eggs, lightly beaten

½ cup whole wheat panko bread crumbs

½ cup roasted red bell peppers, drained and chopped

4 scallions, chopped

2 tablespoons lemon juice

1 tablespoon fat-free mayonnaise

2 teaspoons grated lemon peel

¼ teaspoon hot-pepper sauce

¼ teaspoon salt

3 teaspoons olive oil, divided

1. In a medium bowl, combine the crabmeat, eggs, bread crumbs, bell peppers, scallions, lemon juice, mayonnaise, lemon peel, hot-pepper sauce, and salt. Toss with two forks to mix evenly. Shape into 8 patties.

2. Coat a large nonstick skillet with cooking spray. Add 1½ teaspoons oil and heat over medium heat. Cook 4 patties for 8 minutes, turning once, or until golden brown. Remove to a paper-towel-lined plate. Repeat with the remaining 1½ teaspoons oil and remaining 4 crab patties.

Per serving: 230 calories, 29 g protein, 11 g carbohydrates, 8 g total fat, 2 g saturated fat, 2 g fiber, 750 mg sodium

*serve with 2 grains and 1 vegetable for a complete Phase 2 dinner

Dinner

Salmon Paella

PHASE 2 • **SS** **PMS**

Prep time: 10 minutes • Total time: 1 hour 10 minutes • Makes 4 servings

3 teaspoons canola oil, divided

1 onion, chopped

2 tomatoes, chopped

1 green bell pepper, cut into 1" pieces

2 cloves garlic, chopped

2 teaspoons dried thyme

2 teaspoons fennel seeds

1½ teaspoons smoked paprika

1 cup fat-free, reduced-sodium chicken broth

1 cup white wine

¼ teaspoon ground turmeric

1 cup brown rice

¾ pound skinless salmon fillet, cut into 1½" pieces

¼ teaspoon black pepper, divided

⅛ teaspoon salt

1 cup frozen baby peas, thawed

¼ cup pimiento-stuffed olives, halved

1 tablespoon fresh parsley, chopped

1. Heat 1 teaspoon oil in the pot over medium-high heat. Cook the onion, stirring occasionally, for 5 minutes, or until tender. Add the remaining 1 teaspoon oil. Cook the tomatoes and bell pepper for 4 minutes, or until tender. Cook the garlic, thyme, fennel seeds, and paprika for 1 minute, or until fragrant. Add the broth, wine, and turmeric. Bring to a boil. Stir in the rice. Reduce the heat to medium-low. Cover and simmer for 45 minutes, or until the liquid is absorbed and the rice is tender.

2. Meanwhile, coat a large nonstick pot with cooking spray. Add ½ teaspoon oil and heat over medium-high heat. Season the salmon with ⅛ teaspoon black pepper and the salt. Working in two batches, cook half of the salmon, turning occasionally, for 3 minutes, or until it's opaque. Remove to a plate. Repeat with ½ teaspoon oil and the remaining salmon.

3. Stir the peas, olives, parsley, salmon, and the remaining ⅛ teaspoon black pepper into the rice mixture. Cook for 2 minutes, or until heated through.

Per serving: 470 calories, 27 g protein, 51 g carbohydrates, 13 g total fat, 2 g saturated fat, 7 g fiber, 580 mg sodium

Brown Rice Risotto with Salmon and Asparagus

PHASE 2

Prep time: 10 minutes • Total time: 50 minutes • Makes 4 servings

3 teaspoons canola oil, divided

4 cloves garlic, minced

1 cup short-grain brown rice

1 cup dry white wine

4 cups boiling water, divided

¾ pound skinless salmon fillet, cut into 1½" chunks

⅛ teaspoon + ¼ teaspoon pepper, divided

½ pound asparagus, cut into 1" pieces

1 yellow summer squash, cut in half lengthwise and sliced

4 scallions, sliced

2 tablespoons grated Parmesan cheese

2 tablespoons lemon juice

½ teaspoon salt

1. Coat a large nonstick saucepan with cooking spray. Add 1½ teaspoons oil and heat over medium-high heat. Cook the garlic for 30 seconds, stirring, or until fragrant. Stir in the rice to coat evenly with the oil. Stir in the wine. Cook for 8 minutes, uncovered, or until the wine is absorbed. Stir in 3 cups water. Reduce the heat to medium-low. Cook, stirring occasionally, for 35 to 40 minutes, or until the water is absorbed.

2. Stir in the remaining 1 cup water. Cook for 7 minutes, stirring occasionally.

3. Meanwhile, coat a large, deep nonstick skillet with cooking spray. Add ½ teaspoon oil and heat over medium-high heat. Season the salmon with ⅛ teaspoon pepper. Working in two batches, cook half the salmon for 3 minutes, or until it's opaque. Remove to a plate. Repeat with the remaining salmon.

4. Coat the skillet with cooking spray and heat the remaining 1 teaspoon oil over medium-high heat. Cook the asparagus and squash for 5 minutes, or until tender-crisp. Add to the rice. Gently stir in the salmon. Cook for 2 minutes, or until heated through.

5. Remove from the heat. Gently stir in the scallions, cheese, lemon juice, salt, and the remaining ¼ teaspoon pepper.

Per serving: 430 calories, 26 g protein, 48 g carbohydrates, 12 g total fat, 2 g saturated fat, 6 g fiber, 390 mg sodium

*serve with 1 grain for a complete Phase 2 dinner

Fettuccine with Walnuts

PHASE 2 • SS PMS

Prep time: 10 minutes • Total time: 25 minutes • Makes 4 servings

8 ounces fiber-and-calcium-enriched fettuccine

½ cup walnuts, coarsely chopped

1 tablespoon canola oil

3 cloves garlic, minced

1 cup fat-free half-and-half

1 box (4.4 ounces) light garlic and fine herbs Gourney cheese

1 teaspoon grated lemon peel

¼ teaspoon cracked black pepper

4 cups loosely packed arugula

1 tablespoon fresh parsley, chopped

1. Cook the pasta according to package directions. Drain and reserve ½ cup cooking water.

2. In a large nonstick skillet, cook the walnuts over medium-high heat for 1 to 2 minutes, or until toasted. Remove to a plate.

3. Coat the skillet with cooking spray. Add the oil and heat over low heat. Cook the garlic for 3 minutes, or until softened. Increase the heat to medium-high. Stir in the half-and-half, cheese, lemon peel, and pepper. Cook for 2 minutes, stirring, or until heated through. Stir in the arugula, pasta, and the cooking water. Cook for 1 minute, or until the arugula is wilted. Sprinkle with the walnuts and parsley.

Per serving: 420 calories, 14 g protein, 50 g carbohydrates, 20 g total fat, 2 g saturated fat, 6 g fiber, 250 mg sodium

*serve with 1 protein and ½ vegetable for a complete Phase 2 dinner

Macaroni and Cheese

PHASE 2 • **PMS**

Prep time: 10 minutes • Total time: 30 minutes • Makes 4 servings

8 ounces fiber-and-calcium-enriched elbow pasta

1½ cups fat-free half-and-half

1 package (10 ounces) frozen pureed winter squash, thawed

1½ cups shredded reduced-fat sharp Cheddar cheese

1 small onion, finely chopped

1 tablespoon honey mustard

½ teaspoon salt

¼ teaspoon pepper

2 tablespoons whole wheat panko bread crumbs

2 tablespoons grated Parmesan cheese

1 tablespoon unsalted butter, melted

1 scallion, chopped

1. Preheat the oven to 375°F. Coat a 6-cup baking dish with cooking spray.

2. Prepare the pasta according to package directions.

3. Meanwhile, in a large saucepan over medium heat, combine the half-and-half and squash. Cook for 5 minutes, stirring, or until simmering. Remove from the heat and stir in the Cheddar, onion, mustard, salt, and pepper until the cheese melts. Stir in the pasta. Transfer to the baking dish.

4. In a small bowl, stir together the bread crumbs, Parmesan, butter, and scallion. Sprinkle over the pasta.

5. Bake for 20 minutes, or until golden brown and bubbling.

Per serving: 480 calories, 25 g protein, 65 g carbohydrates, 13 g total fat, 7 g saturated fat, 3 g fiber, 760 mg sodium

*uses extra 1 dairy

**serve with 2 proteins and 1 vegetable for a complete Phase 2 dinner

Dinner

Eggplant Parmesan

PHASE 2 • **SS** **PMS**

Prep time: 10 minutes • Total time: 40 minutes • Makes 4 servings

1 tablespoon canola oil

1 onion, chopped

3 teaspoons dried Italian seasoning, divided

1 can (28 ounces) no-salt-added crushed tomatoes

1½ cups whole wheat panko bread crumbs

¼ cup grated Parmesan cheese

1 teaspoon garlic powder

¼ teaspoon pepper

2 omega-3-enriched eggs

2 eggplants (1 pound each), sliced ¼" thick

1½ cups shredded reduced-fat mozzarella cheese

1. Heat the oil in a large nonstick skillet over medium-high heat. Cook the onion for 8 minutes, stirring occasionally, or until softened. Stir in 1½ teaspoons Italian seasoning and cook for 30 seconds, or until fragrant. Add the tomatoes and bring to a boil. Reduce the heat to medium-low. Cover and cook, for 10 minutes, stirring occasionally, or until slightly thickened.

2. Meanwhile, preheat the oven to 425°F. Coat 2 baking sheets and a 13" × 9" baking dish with cooking spray.

3. In a shallow bowl, stir together the bread crumbs, Parmesan, garlic powder, pepper, and the remaining 1½ teaspoons Italian seasoning. Whisk the eggs in a shallow bowl. One at a time, dip the eggplant slices into the egg and then into the bread crumb mixture to coat evenly. Place on the baking sheets. Coat with cooking spray.

4. Bake for 15 minutes, turning once and coating with cooking spray, or until crisp and golden brown.

5. Spoon 1 cup tomato sauce in the bottom of the baking dish. Top with half of the eggplant slices and 1½ cups sauce. Repeat the layering with the remaining eggplant slices and remaining sauce. Sprinkle with the mozzarella.

6. Cover and bake for 20 minutes, or until the cheese is bubbly.

Per serving: 400 calories, 24 g protein, 46 g carbohydrates, 15 g total fat, 6 g saturated fat, 12 g fiber, 440 mg sodium

*uses extra 1 dairy

**serve with 2 proteins and 1 grain for a complete Phase 2 dinner

Whole Wheat Gnocchi with Broccoli Raab

PHASE 1 OR 2 • SS PMS

Prep time: 10 minutes • Total time: 30 minutes • Makes 4 servings

1 package (1.1 pounds) prepared shelf-stable whole wheat gnocchi

3 teaspoons canola oil, divided

1 onion, chopped

1 pound broccoli raab, trimmed and coarsely chopped

3 cloves garlic, sliced

1 tablespoon fresh rosemary, chopped

1 cup fat-free, reduced-sodium chicken broth

1 can (14.5 ounces) no-salt-added diced tomatoes

1 can (15 ounces) no-salt-added white beans, rinsed and drained

$\frac{1}{4}$ teaspoon pepper

3 tablespoons grated Parmesan cheese

1 tablespoon lemon juice

1. Prepare the gnocchi according to package directions

2. Coat a large nonstick skillet with cooking spray. Heat 1½ teaspoons oil over medium-high heat. Cook the onion for 4 minutes, stirring, or until tender. Heat the remaining 1½ teaspoons oil over medium-high heat. Cook the broccoli raab, garlic, and rosemary for 2 minutes, stirring, or until slightly softened. Add the broth. Reduce the heat to medium-low. Cover and cook for 7 minutes, or until the broccoli raab is tender. Stir in the tomatoes, beans, and pepper. Bring to a simmer. Stir in the gnocchi, cheese, and lemon juice. Cover and cook for 3 minutes, or until the cheese melts and the sauce is bubbling.

Per serving: 420 calories, 17 g protein, 76 g carbohydrates, 6 g total fat, 1 g saturated fat, 10 g fiber, 900 mg sodium

*substitute 3–4 tablespoons water for the oil for Phase 1

Bulgur Lentil Pilaf with Apple

PHASE 1 OR 2 • SS PMS

Prep time: 10 minutes • Total time: 30 minutes • Makes 4 servings

1 can (14.5 ounces) fat-free, reduced-sodium chicken broth

1½ cups bulgur wheat

1 cup apple juice

1 tablespoon canola oil

2 carrots, chopped

1 red bell pepper, cut into 1" pieces

1 small green apple, chopped

1 small red onion, chopped

1 can (15 ounces) lentils, drained and rinsed

1 tablespoon fresh parsley, chopped

1 tablespoon grated lemon peel

1 tablespoon lemon juice

⅛ teaspoon black pepper

1. In a small saucepan, combine the broth, bulgur, and apple juice. Bring to a boil over high heat. Reduce the heat to medium-low. Cover and cook for 15 minutes, or until the liquid is absorbed and the bulgur is tender. Remove from the heat and fluff with a fork.

2. Coat a large nonstick skillet with cooking spray. Heat the oil over medium-high heat. Cook the carrots, bell pepper, apple, and onion for 5 minutes, stirring, or until tender. Remove from the heat. Stir in the lentils, parsley, lemon peel, lemon juice, black pepper, and bulgur.

Per serving: 370 calories, 14 g protein, 73 g carbohydrates, 4 g total fat, 1 g saturated fat, 20 g fiber, 390 mg sodium

*substitute 3–4 tablespoons water for the oil for Phase 1

Sesame-Crusted Tofu over Noodles

PHASE 2 • SS PMS

Prep time: 20 minutes • Total time: 35 minutes • Makes 4 servings

8 ounces fiber-and-calcium-enriched spaghetti

¼ cup sesame seeds

4 teaspoons cornstarch, divided

½ teaspoon salt, divided

1 package (14 ounces) extra-firm water-packed lite tofu, drained

3 teaspoons canola oil, divided

2 tablespoons chopped fresh ginger

2 cloves garlic, minced

1¼ pounds broccoli, trimmed and cut into florets

2 carrots, sliced

¼ teaspoon red-pepper flakes

1 cup orange juice

2 tablespoons reduced-sodium soy sauce

1 teaspoon toasted sesame oil

1. Prepare the pasta according to package directions. Drain the pasta, reserving 1 cup cooking water. Set aside.

2. On a plate, combine the sesame seeds, 2 teaspoons cornstarch, and ¼ teaspoon salt. Cut the tofu lengthwise into 8 thin slices. Pat dry with a paper towel. Press both sides of the tofu into the sesame mixture.

3. Coat a large nonstick skillet with cooking spray. Add 1½ teaspoons oil and heat over medium-high heat. Cook the tofu for 6 minutes, turning once, or until golden brown. Transfer to a plate. Cover to keep warm.

4. Wipe out the skillet and coat with cooking spray. Add the remaining 1½ teaspoons oil. Cook the ginger and garlic over medium-high heat for 1 minute. Cook the broccoli, carrots, pepper flakes, and the remaining ¼ teaspoon salt, stirring, for 4 to 5 minutes, or until the broccoli is tender-crisp.

5. Place the remaining 2 teaspoons cornstarch in a bowl. Whisk in the orange juice, soy sauce, and reserved cooking water until smooth. Add to the skillet. Bring to a boil over high heat. Cook for 2 minutes, stirring, or until the sauce is thickened. Toss in the pasta and sesame oil. Serve with the tofu.

Per serving: 480 calories, 22 g protein, 69 g carbohydrates, 13 g total fat, 1 g saturated fat, 8 g fiber, 610 mg sodium

Dinner

Chocolate 'n' Peanut Banana

PHASE 2 • **PMS**

Prep time: 5 minutes • Total time: 5 minutes • Makes 1 serving

2 chocolate wafer cookies, crushed

2 tablespoons chopped unsalted peanuts

1 small banana, diagonally cut into 6 slices

In a shallow bowl, stir together the cookies and nuts. Press both sides of the banana slices into the mixture to coat.

Per serving: 240 calories, 6 g protein, 40 g carbohydrates, 10 g total fat, 2 g saturated fat, 4 g fiber, 95 mg sodium

*serve with ½ dairy for a complete Phase 2 midmorning snack

Fresh Fruit with Lime Yogurt Dip

PHASE 2 • **PMS**

Prep time: 10 minutes • Total time: 10 minutes • Makes 1 serving

½ cup 0% vanilla Greek yogurt

½ teaspoon lime juice

½ teaspoon grated lime peel

½ cup fresh pineapple chunks

1 kiwifruit, cut into chunks

In a small bowl, whisk together the yogurt, lime juice, and lime peel. Serve as a dip with the pineapple and kiwifruit.

Per serving: 170 calories, 12 g protein, 31 g carbohydrates, 0 g total fat, 0 g saturated fat, 4 g fiber, 55 mg sodium

Café Latte

Prep time: 5 minutes • Total time: 10 minutes • Makes 1 serving

1 cup fat-free milk
½ cup strong brewed coffee
2 teaspoons sugar

⅛ teaspoon ground cinnamon + a dash for garnish

1. In a 2-cup microwaveable measuring cup, whisk together the milk, coffee, sugar, and ⅛ teaspoon cinnamon. Microwave on medium power for 3 to 5 minutes, or until steaming.

2. Transfer the mixture to a blender. Blend for 30 seconds, or until frothy. Pour into a large mug and sprinkle with cinnamon.

Per serving: 120 calories, 9 g protein, 21 g carbohydrates, 0 g total fat, 0 g saturated fat, 0 g fiber, 110 mg sodium

*uses extra ½ dairy

**serve with 1 fruit for a complete Phase 2 midmorning snack

Snacks: Midmorning

Baked Stuffed Apple

PHASE 2 • **PMS**

Prep time: 5 minutes • Total time: 10 minutes • Makes 1 serving

1 Granny Smith apple, cored

1 teaspoon sugar

¼ teaspoon apple pie spice

1 tablespoon chopped walnuts

1 tablespoon golden raisins

1 tablespoon water

½ cup 0% vanilla Greek yogurt

1. Place the apple in a microwaveable dish. Sprinkle with the sugar and apple pie spice. Stuff the walnuts and raisins into the cavity. Add the water to the dish and cover with plastic wrap.

2. Microwave on high power for 2 to 3 minutes, or until tender. Serve with the yogurt.

Per serving: 270 calories, 13 g protein, 48 g carbohydrates, 5 g total fat, 1 g saturated fat, 5 g fiber, 55 mg sodium

Chocolate Mint Parfait

Prep time: 5 minutes • Total time: 5 minutes • Makes 1 serving

½ cup fat-free ricotta cheese
1 spearmint Starlight Mint candy, crushed
1 drop green food coloring

2 tablespoons frozen fat-free whipped topping, thawed
1 chocolate wafer cookie, crushed

In a small bowl, stir together the cheese, candy, and food coloring. Fold in the whipped topping. Spoon into a parfait glass. Top with the cookie.

Per serving: 150 calories, 16 g protein, 19 g carbohydrates, 1 g total fat, 0 g saturated fat, 0 g fiber, 210 mg sodium

*serve with ½ fruit for a complete Phase 1 midafternoon snack

Crave-Reducing Shake

PHASE 1 • SS PMS

Prep time: 5 minutes • Total time: 5 minutes • Makes 1 serving

½ large frozen banana, cut into 1" chunks
½ cup 0% vanilla Greek yogurt

½ cup fat-free milk
1 teaspoon ground flaxseed
1 teaspoon mini chocolate chips

1. In a blender or a food processor, combine the banana, yogurt, milk, and flaxseed. Blend or process for 1 minute, or until smooth. Stir in the chips.

2. Drink immediately or transfer to a freezer-proof container. Place in the freezer for up to 3 days. Thaw in the refrigerator for several hours.

Per serving: 220 calories, 16 g protein, 34 g carbohydrates, 3 g total fat, 1 g saturated fat, 3 g fiber, 105 mg sodium

Snacks: Midafternoon

Apple Cinnamon Yogurt

PHASE 1 • **SS** **PMS**

Prep time: 5 minutes • Total time: 5 minutes • Makes 1 serving

1 cup 0% vanilla Greek yogurt

1 small apple, chopped

½ teaspoon ground flaxseed

⅛ teaspoon ground cinnamon

In a small bowl, stir together the yogurt, apple, flaxseed, and cinnamon.

Per serving: 240 calories, 22 g protein, 38 g carbohydrates, 1 g total fat, 0 g saturated fat, 4 g fiber, 100 mg sodium

Watermelon Frappé

PHASE 2 • **SS** **PMS**

Prep time: 5 minutes • Total time: 5 minutes • Makes 1 serving

5 ounces (1 cup) watermelon cubes

½ cup 0% vanilla Greek yogurt

1 tablespoon fresh mint, chopped

1 teaspoon lemon juice

¼ teaspoon ground ginger

In a blender or a food processor, combine the watermelon, yogurt, mint, lemon juice, and ginger. Blend or process for 1 minute, or until smooth.

Per serving: 130 calories, 12 g protein, 21 g carbohydrates, 0 g total fat, 0 g saturated fat, 1 g fiber, 55 mg sodium

*uses extra ½ fruit

Orange-Scented Ricotta with Chocolate Crunchies

PHASE 2 • **SS** **PMS**

Prep time: 5 minutes • Total time: 5 minutes • Makes 1 serving

½ cup fat-free ricotta cheese

1 tablespoon orange juice

1 teaspoon grated orange peel

½ teaspoon sugar

2 chocolate wafer cookies, coarsely crushed

In a small bowl, stir together the cheese, orange juice, orange peel, and sugar. Spoon into a parfait glass. Sprinkle with the cookies.

Per serving: 160 calories, 17 g protein, 20 g carbohydrates, 2 g total fat, 1 g saturated fat, 1 g fiber, 250 mg sodium

Carrot Cake Smoothie

PHASE 2 • **SS** **PMS**

Prep time: 5 minutes • Total time: 5 minutes • Makes 1 serving

¾ cup canned sliced carrots, drained

¾ cup 0% vanilla Greek yogurt

⅓ cup canned crushed pineapple, in juice

¼ cup fat-free milk

¼ teaspoon ground pumpkin pie spice

3 ice cubes

In a blender or a food processor, combine the carrots, yogurt, pineapple, milk, pumpkin pie spice, and ice. Blend or process for 30 seconds, or until thickened.

Per serving: 220 calories, 19 g protein, 35 g carbohydrates, 0 g total fat, 0 g saturated fat, 2 g fiber, 370 mg sodium

*uses extra ½ fruit

Chocolate-Malt Ricotta

PHASE 2 • **SS** **PMS**

Prep time: 5 minutes • Total time: 5 minutes • Makes 1 serving

½ cup fat-free ricotta cheese

2 teaspoons chocolate malted-milk powder

1 teaspoon unsweetened cocoa powder

½ teaspoon sugar

2 tablespoons frozen fat-free whipped topping, thawed

In a bowl, stir together the cheese, malted-milk powder, cocoa powder, and sugar. Fold in the whipped topping.

Per serving: 130 calories, 17 g protein, 13 g carbohydrates, 1 g total fat, 0 g saturated fat, 0 g fiber, 170 mg sodium

Decadent Hot Chocolate

PHASE 2 • **SS** **PMS**

Prep time: 5 minutes • Total time: 5 minutes • Makes 2 servings

2 cups fat-free milk

⅓ cup unsweetened cocoa powder

1 tablespoon cornstarch

1½ teaspoons sugar

In a microwaveable mixing bowl, whisk together the milk, cocoa powder, cornstarch, and sugar (mixture will be lumpy). Microwave on high power for 2 minutes, or until hot. Whisk for 10 seconds.

Per serving: 190 calories, 11 g protein, 33 g carbohydrates, 2 g total fat, 0 g saturated fat, 3 g fiber, 105 mg sodium

Cheesy Lemon-Pepper Dip

PHASE 2 • **SS** **PMS**

Prep time: 5 minutes • Total time: 5 minutes • Makes 1 serving

1 cup fat-free cottage cheese
½ teaspoon salt-free lemon-pepper
seasoning

½ cup baby carrots
½ cup snow peas

In a bowl, stir together the cottage cheese and lemon-pepper seasoning. Serve with the carrots and snow peas for dipping.

Per serving: 140 calories, 17 g protein, 18 g carbohydrates, 0 g total fat, 0 g saturated fat, 2 g fiber, 510 mg sodium

*serve with ½ dairy for a complete Phase 2 midafternoon snack

Berry Chocolate Frozen-Yogurt Pops

PHASE 2 • **SS** **PMS**

**Prep time: 5 minutes • Total time: 5 minutes + 6 hours freezing time •
Makes 4 servings**

1 cup fresh or frozen strawberries or
raspberries
1 cup 0% vanilla Greek yogurt

1 tablespoon sugar
1 tablespoon mini chocolate chips

1. In a food processor or a blender, combine the berries, yogurt, and sugar. Process or blend for 2 minutes, or until smooth.

2. Divide the mixture among 4 freezer-pop molds (3 ounces each). Divide the chips among the molds. Stir with a knife to incorporate and burst any air pockets. Insert the sticks.

3. Place in the freezer for 6 hours, or until solid.

Per serving: 80 calories, 6 g protein, 13 g carbohydrates, 1 g total fat, 1 g saturated fat, 1 g fiber, 25 mg sodium

*uses extra ½ fruit

Gingersnap Oatmeal

Prep time: 5 minutes • Total time: 5 minutes • Makes 1 serving

¼ cup quick-cooking rolled oats

1 gingersnap cookie, coarsely crushed

Cook the oats according to package directions. Sprinkle with the cookie.

Per serving: 110 calories, 3 g protein, 19 g carbohydrates, 3 g total fat, 1 g saturated fat, 2 g fiber, 45 mg sodium

*serve with ½ dairy for a complete Phase 1 evening snack

Parmesan Popcorn

PHASE 1

Prep time: 5 minutes • Total time: 5 minutes • Makes 1 serving

3 cups air-popped popcorn
Butter-flavored cooking spray

1 tablespoon grated Parmesan cheese

Place the popcorn in a large bowl. Coat generously with cooking spray. Toss in the cheese.

Per serving: 110 calories, 5 g protein, 19 g carbohydrates, 3 g total fat, 1 g saturated fat, 3 g fiber, 80 mg sodium

*serve with ½ dairy for a complete Phase 1 evening snack

Lemon Almond Cheesecake Parfait

PHASE 2 • **SS** **PMS**

Prep time: 5 minutes • Total time: 5 minutes • Makes 1 serving

½ cup fat-free ricotta cheese
½ teaspoon sugar
½ teaspoon grated lemon peel
2 tablespoons frozen fat-free
   whipped topping, thawed

½ cup raspberries
1 small almond biscotti, coarsely
   crushed

In a small bowl, stir together the cheese, sugar, and lemon peel. Fold in the whipped topping. Spoon into a small parfait glass and top with raspberries and biscotti.

Per serving: 230 calories, 18 g protein, 33 g carbohydrates, 4 g total fat, 2 g saturated fat, 0 g fiber, 210 mg sodium

Chocolate Pudding

PHASE 2 • **SS** **PMS**

Prep time: 5 minutes • Total time: 10 minutes • Makes 2 servings

2 cups fat-free milk
3 tablespoons cornstarch
1 ounce unsweetened chocolate,
   chopped

1½ tablespoons sugar
½ teaspoon instant coffee powder
⅛ teaspoon salt
½ teaspoon vanilla extract

1. In a medium saucepan, whisk together the milk, cornstarch, chocolate, sugar, coffee powder, and salt. Cook over medium heat for 5 minutes, whisking occasionally, or until the mixture boils. Reduce the heat to medium-low. Cook for 3 minutes, whisking, or until thickened.

2. Remove from the heat and stir in the vanilla.

Per serving: 260 calories, 10 g protein, 37 g carbohydrates, 7 g total fat, 5 g saturated fat, 0 g fiber, 250 mg sodium

*serve with 1 grain and ½ fruit for a complete Phase 2 evening snack

Chai Sugar Pita Chips

PHASE 2 • **PMS**

Prep time: 5 minutes • Total time: 15 minutes • Makes 1 serving

1 whole wheat pita (4" diameter), cut
  into sixths
  Butter-flavored cooking spray

¼ teaspoon sugar
¼ teaspoon ground chai spice

1. Preheat the oven to 350°F. Place the pita on a small baking sheet. Coat with cooking spray.

2. In a small bowl, stir together the sugar and chai. Sprinkle evenly over the pita.

3. Bake for 10 minutes, or until crisp.

Per serving: 80 calories, 3 g protein, 17 g carbohydrates, 1 g total fat, 0 g saturated fat, 2 g fiber, 150 mg sodium

*serve with 1 dairy and ½ fruit for a complete Phase 2 evening snack

Toasted Coconut and Banana Crepes

PHASE 2 • **SS** **PMS**

Prep time: 5 minutes • Total time: 5 minutes • Makes 1 serving

¾ cup 0% vanilla Greek yogurt
2 tablespoons flaked coconut,
  toasted
½ teaspoon ground flaxseed

½ teaspoon coconut extract
½ banana, sliced
2 crepes (7" or 8" diameter)

In a bowl, stir together the yogurt, coconut, flaxseed, and coconut extract. Divide the yogurt mixture and banana among the crepes. Roll up.

Per serving: 300 calories, 19 g protein, 41 g carbohydrates, 6 g total fat, 5 g saturated fat, 3 g fiber, 180 mg sodium

Strawberry Cream-Cheese Sandwich

PHASE 2

Prep time: 5 minutes • Total time: 5 minutes • Makes 1 serving

2 tablespoons fat-free cream cheese, at room temperature

¼ teaspoon grated lemon peel

2 slices very thin whole wheat sandwich bread

2 strawberries, sliced

In a small bowl, stir together the cream cheese and lemon peel. Spread on 1 slice of the bread. Top with the strawberries and remaining slice of bread.

Per serving: 180 calories, 11 g protein, 27 g carbohydrates, 3 g total fat, 0 g saturated fat, 5 g fiber, 390 mg sodium

*serve with 1 dairy for a complete Phase 2 evening snack

Snacks: Evening

Fig Almond Biscotti

Prep time: 15 minutes • Total time: 1 hour 5 minutes • Makes 24 cookies

¾ cup whole wheat flour

½ cup unbleached or all-purpose flour

½ cup ground flaxseed

¼ cup firmly packed light brown sugar

1 teaspoon baking powder

2 omega-3-enriched eggs

¼ cup fat-free milk

2½ tablespoons canola oil

2 tablespoons honey

1 teaspoon almond extract

1 bag (6 ounces) Calimyrna dried figs, quartered

¼ cup + 2 tablespoons coarsely chopped unblanched sliced almonds, toasted

1. Preheat the oven to 350°F. Coat a baking sheet with cooking spray.

2. In a large bowl, whisk together the flours, flaxseed, sugar, and baking powder.

3. In a bowl, whisk together the eggs, milk, oil, honey, and almond extract. Using a wooden spoon, stir the liquid mixture into the dry ingredients just until the dough begins to come together. Add the figs and ¼ cup of the almonds. With floured hands, knead until the dough is well blended.

4. Place the dough on a long sheet of plastic wrap and shape by hand into a flattened 12"-long log. Lift the wrap to invert the dough onto the baking sheet, discarding the wrap. Sprinkle with the remaining 2 tablespoons almonds. Press lightly to adhere.

5. Bake for 25 minutes, or until lightly browned. Transfer to a cutting board to cool for 10 minutes. Leave the oven on. With a serrated knife, cut diagonally into 24 slices. Arrange the slices, cut side down, on the baking sheet.

6. Bake for 15 minutes, or until crisp. Cool on the pan on a rack for 5 minutes. Remove to the rack and cool completely. Store in an airtight container.

Per cookie: 90 calories, 2 g protein, 13 g carbohydrates, 4 g total fat, 0 g saturated fat, 2 g fiber, 25 mg sodium

*serve with 1 dairy and ½ fruit for a complete Phase 2 evening snack

S'mores

PHASE 2

Prep time: 5 minutes • Total time: 10 minutes • Makes 1 serving

1 whole graham cracker, broken in
half
2 large marshmallows

1 tablespoon bittersweet chocolate
chips

1. Position a rack in the upper third of a toaster oven. Preheat the broiler.

2. Place the graham cracker halves on a small baking sheet. Top each with 1 marshmallow. Broil for 2 minutes, or until the marshmallows are golden brown. Place on a plate.

3. Meanwhile, in a small microwaveable bowl, microwave the chips for 10 seconds (watch carefully so they don't burn). Drizzle the marshmallows with the chocolate.

Per serving: 210 calories, 3 g protein, 40 g carbohydrates, 6 g total fat, 3 g saturated fat, 1 g fiber, 150 mg sodium

*serve with 1 dairy and ½ fruit for a complete Phase 2 evening snack

Honey-Scented Peaches 'n' Cream

PHASE 2 • SS PMS

Prep time: 5 minutes • Total time: 5 minutes • Makes 1 serving

1 cup 0% vanilla Greek yogurt
1 small peach, sliced

⅓ cup low-fat granola
½ teaspoon honey

In a small bowl, layer the yogurt, peach, and granola. Drizzle with the honey.

Per serving: 330 calories, 25 g protein, 54 g carbohydrates, 2 g total fat, 0 g saturated fat, 3 g fiber, 170 mg sodium

Mini Chocolate Chipwich

Prep time: 5 minutes • Total time: 1 hour 5 minutes • Makes 1 serving

¼ cup frozen fat-free whipped
   topping, thawed

1 teaspoon mini chocolate chips

4 mini chocolate rice cakes

1. In a small bowl, stir together the whipped topping and chocolate chips. Spread evenly over 2 rice cakes. Gently cover with the remaining rice cakes.

2. Freeze for at least 1 hour.

Per serving: 90 calories, 1 g protein, 17 g carbohydrates, 2 g total fat, 1 g saturated fat, 0 g fiber, 35 mg sodium

*serve with ½ fruit and 1 dairy for a complete Phase 2 evening snack

Snacks: Evening

Raspberry Tiramisu

PHASE 2 • **SS** **PMS**

Prep time: 10 minutes • Total time: 15 minutes • Makes 1 serving

4 soft ladyfingers

½ tablespoon coffee liqueur or strong coffee

½ cup fat-free ricotta cheese

1 teaspoon instant espresso powder

1 teaspoon sugar

½ teaspoon vanilla extract

2 tablespoons frozen fat-free whipped topping, thawed

½ cup raspberries

1. Brush the ladyfingers with the liqueur or coffee. Line the sides of a small parfait glass with the ladyfingers.

2. In a small bowl, stir together the cheese, espresso powder, sugar, and vanilla. Let stand for 5 minutes for the espresso powder to dissolve. Fold in the whipped topping. Spoon half of the mixture into the glass. Top with half of the raspberries. Repeat with the remaining cheese mixture and raspberries.

Per serving: 260 calories, 18 g protein, 42 g carbohydrates, 2 g total fat, 0 g saturated fat, 0 g fiber, 200 mg sodium

Snacks: Evening

Toasted Almond and Chocolate Parfait

PHASE 2 • **SS** **PMS**

Prep time: 5 minutes • Total time: 5 minutes • Makes 1 serving

1 cup 0% vanilla Greek yogurt
¼ teaspoon almond extract
4 strawberries, sliced

2 chocolate wafer cookies, coarsely crushed
1 tablespoon unblanched sliced almonds, toasted

In a small bowl, stir together the yogurt and almond extract. In a parfait glass, layer half of the yogurt mixture, strawberries, and cookies. Repeat with the layering. Sprinkle with the almonds.

Per serving: 280 calories, 24 g protein, 34 g carbohydrates, 5 g total fat, 1 g saturated fat, 2 g fiber, 190 mg sodium

Blueberry Fluff with Ginger Crunchies

PHASE 2 • **SS** **PMS**

Prep time: 5 minutes • Total time: 5 minutes • Makes 1 serving

½ cup fat-free ricotta cheese
½ teaspoon sugar
¼ teaspoon ground ginger

2 tablespoons frozen fat-free whipped topping, thawed
½ cup blueberries
2 gingersnap cookies, crushed

In a medium bowl, stir together the cheese, sugar, and ginger. Fold in the whipped topping. Spoon into a small parfait glass. Top with the blueberries and cookies.

Per serving: 210 calories, 17 g protein, 31 g carbohydrates, 3 g total fat, 1 g saturated fat, 2 g fiber, 210 mg sodium

Rice Pudding

PHASE 2 • **PMS**

Prep time: 5 minutes • Total time: 25 minutes • Makes 2 servings

1¼ cups fat-free milk

½ cup instant brown rice

½ cup water

1 tablespoon + 1 teaspoon sugar

1 tablespoon dried currants

½ teaspoon ground cinnamon

¼ teaspoon salt

1½ teaspoons vanilla extract

In a heavy saucepan, combine the milk, rice, water, sugar, currants, cinnamon, and salt. Cook over medium heat for 5 minutes, stirring, or until the mixture simmers. Reduce the heat to low. Cover and simmer, for 20 minutes, stirring occasionally, or until the rice is very tender. Stir in the vanilla. Serve warm or refrigerate to serve cold.

Per serving: 280 calories, 9 g protein, 56 g carbohydrates, 2 g total fat, 0 g saturated fat, 3 g fiber, 65 mg sodium

*serve with ½ fruit for a complete Phase 2 evening snack

Snacks: Evening

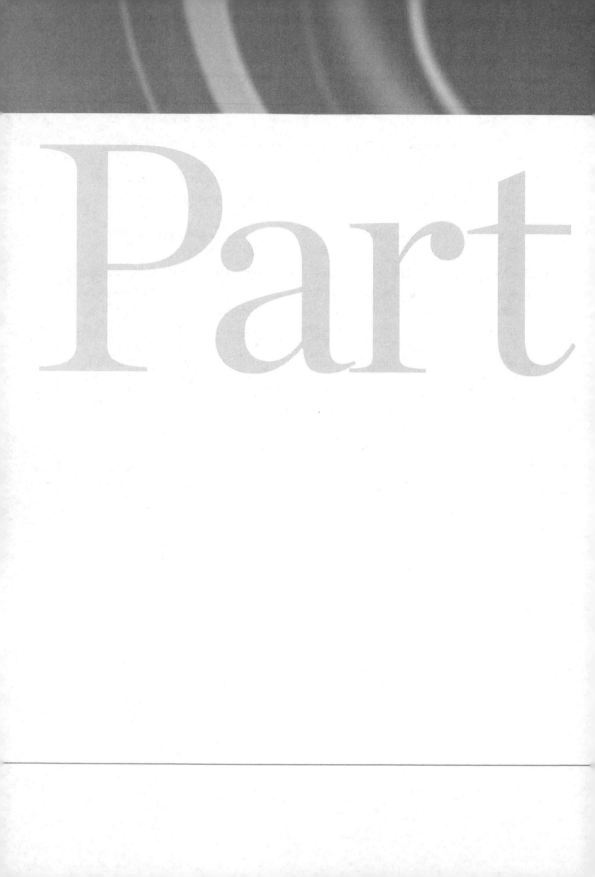

Part

III

The
Perfect Timing
Workouts

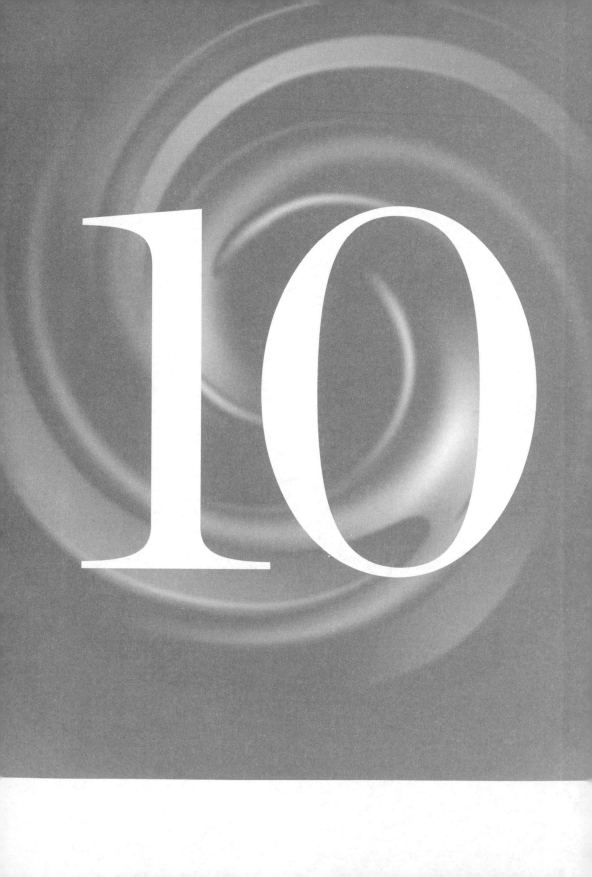

The Best Time to Burn Belly Fat

You've learned how to improve both your sleep and your eating habits by working with, not against, the natural rhythms of your body. Now we'll explore how to exercise in the best possible way to rev your metabolism and burn belly fat fast. Whether you actually look forward to working out or, like so many of us, you grumble every time you lace up your sneakers, getting your exercise in sync with your circadian rhythm can make your workouts more effective, more satisfying, and even fun.

Not surprisingly, a lot of the research on the optimal time of the day to work out has been done with elite athletes—Olympic competitors or players on professional sports teams. It makes sense. More than anyone, they need to optimize their performance. But we can use those results to find out when you'd get the most benefit from moving your body.

If you've never been a lover of exercise, then this chapter is for you. You'll find out why it's always been a struggle for you to get moving (you were probably forcing your body to move when it wasn't ready), and you'll see just how easy it is. Also, the exercises are divided into 20-minute sessions—so no matter how busy you are, you can fit this workout plan into any schedule!

Wake Up with a Morning Walk

We're going to be honest here: This is the part of the workout that our panelists didn't love so much, at least in the beginning. But there's a huge health, fitness, and circadian rhythm bonus to waking up and walking out the door first thing in the morning—and we're only asking for about 20 minutes.

Doing some cardio before breakfast can stimulate your body to burn fat more efficiently. That's what Belgian researchers found in a study published in the *Journal of Physiology* in 2010. They put three groups of subjects on a high-calorie, high-fat diet. One group did not exercise at all. The other two groups cycled or ran for 90 minutes (twice a week) or an hour (twice a week), with one group exercising before breakfast, the other after they ate.

At the end of 6 weeks, the no-exercise group had gained 6 pounds on average, and the exercise-after-breakfast subjects gained about 3. But the group that worked out before breakfast gained *less than a pound* on average. So even though they ate the same high-fat, not-so-great-for-you breakfast every morning, the pre-breakfast exercisers barely gained any weight while those in the two other groups gained!

There was another important benefit to exercising before eating: Only the exercise-before-breakfast group did not develop insulin resistance (a condition that can lead to diabetes), whereas those in the other two groups did. Researchers believe that several factors help explain these results. For one thing, the group that worked out before breakfast had higher levels of a protein that helps regulate insulin sensitivity. Also, when you exercise before you eat, it encourages your body to burn a greater percentage of fat for fuel, rather than the carbs from your meal.

So if you can get up and go before breakfast each morning, you can possibly help blunt any effect of your morning meal (although the ones you'll be eating will be much healthier) and burn more fat. That's pretty good incentive to wake up and slip on your sneakers before breakfast. But remember, it doesn't have to be walking; that's just the easiest. Whatever you like to do—run, bike, climb the step machine—is fine; just try to do it before breakfast.

There are other reasons to take a walk or a run before you eat in the morning. Exercising in the morning will make you more alert, which can be a boon if you're an owl trying to be more like a lark. You'll get a nice mood boost from your workout, particularly if you exercise outdoors. And exposure to natural light will help you wake up and kick your circadian wake-up rhythm into high gear.

The Right Time to Tone

It's no coincidence that late afternoon and evening are when many track-and-field world records are set; that's the time of day when the heart and lungs work most efficiently. Many dimensions of athleticism peak in late afternoon or early evening—you're stronger, faster, and generally more able at that time. That's because your body temperature is peaking, and when muscles are warmer, they're more powerful and less prone to injury. Furthermore, we're less likely to get hurt because our tendons and ligaments are more elastic in the late afternoon or evening. Ditto for our joints.

But there's another, bigger benefit to exercising in the late afternoon and evening hours: more muscle in less time. A European study cited by Michael Smolensky in his book, *The Body Clock Guide to Better Health,* found that subjects who strength-trained in the evening showed 20 percent greater muscle strength than a group that trained in the morning. And in a 2009 study in Finland, participants in a 20-week study who worked out in the afternoon built 3.5 percent more lean muscle, as compared with 2.7 percent for a group that exercised in the morning.

It makes sense that your muscles will respond better to strength training at the time of day when they are at their best. Your body operates at its most efficient in the afternoon and early evening, according to *Keeping Time with Your Body Clock,* a book by U.K. researchers who specialize in circadian rhythms and exercise. And that means better results.

This could also help explain why your body may have screamed and moaned (or maybe it was just your brain) during previous attempts if you tried to do

Stretch After You Tone

A lot of people get loose and limber before they work out, but research shows that stretching works better if you wait until after you've done your lean-muscle-building moves. Stretching after a weights workout can boost the effectiveness of a strength-training session by a whopping 20 percent, according to Wayne Westcott, PhD, exercise science research director, Quincy College in Quincy, Massachusetts, and his associate Rita La Rosa Loud, exercise science instructor, Quincy College, both of whom created the strength-training program for this book. Further proof that by exercising at certain times in your cycle you can maximize your results!

CAN'T WALK IN THE MORNING?

If despite your best efforts, the before-breakfast mini-workout just isn't happening, don't despair. You'll actually see great cardio results in the afternoon and early evening hours as well, for the same reason—your body is at its most efficient. It's just that the potential benefits of a pre-breakfast walk or other cardio are so amazing that we couldn't resist telling you about it!

your resistance training at another time of day. It just wasn't ready to do it yet. When you exercise at the peak time of your body's natural daily cycle, it will seem easier, be more enjoyable, and as we said, you'll see better results.

And by late afternoon to early evening, we mean around 4:00 to 8:00 for normal 9-to-5ers out there. That gives you plenty of opportunity to fit it into your schedule.

Shift workers, never fear. Our panelist Erin did her "afternoon" workout when she got off work at midnight. Again, it's not the time of day that you exercise that counts, but rather the time of day that's best for your cycle. So for you, doing a 1:30 a.m. resistance workout is the same as someone who works 9 to 5 hitting the gym at 6:00 p.m.

Syncing Up Your Workouts

Just as eating at the same time every day can reset your natural clock and help you eat more healthfully, so too can exercising at the same general time help push your circadian rhythm to a happier place. Your body comes to expect it—dare we say *crave* it, as some of our panelists said—so that you start to look forward to working out. And making exercise part of your daily routine will also help ensure that you'll stick with it.

Get Moving

If your energy falters at another time of the day, a little exercise can give you a boost. Add a quick walk—outdoors if you can—after lunch, if your energy and alertness begin to sag in the afternoon. Just 10 minutes will reinvigorate you.

We've devised a program that won't take big chunks out of your day but will yield big results. You'll do 20 minutes of cardio in the morning to kick off your day with high energy, plus 20 minutes (or less!) of strength training four times a week, in the late afternoon or evening, when your body is most receptive to building lean muscle.

On the days that you're not strength training, you can add another cardio session or some yoga poses; we have five to energize you, and five to relax you (see page 308).

The Big 4 flat-belly moves. Want a bikini-worthy body? These four moves have been scientifically proven to get you the best belly-busting results anywhere (see page 293). Do this workout twice a week (tack one onto another short workout and use one of your free nights for the other). And once you've got the Big 4 down, you'll be ready to try our challenging Super-Lean Workout (see page 298); substitute it for one of your regular-strength workouts.

The best part: As you'll see, these moves are basic and can be done with equipment or without, so you can use whatever you have around the house. There's no pain, only big gains in this workout plan!

Exercising with the Seasons

So far, we've been talking clock—parsing the 24-hour day to make the most of it by eating, sleeping, and exercising at the best times. Now we're going to think on a bigger scale—the 12 months that add up to a year. Such larger rhythms, as we've learned, are called infradian—the ones that occur less frequently than once a day. Let's take a look at how the seasons can affect our exercise plan.

As the seasons change, your body observes the changes in a variety of ways, though you may not be aware of them as they're happening. It's no wonder that you sweat more in summer; wintertime sweat is less profuse and saltier, too. Basal (resting) metabolism rises in winter to keep our bodies warm. Follicle-stimulating hormone peaks twice a year, in February and October, as does testosterone, in summer and winter. Cortisol and insulin peak in wintertime, when bone mineral density is lowest. These bodily changes occur for a variety of reasons that are not fully understood, but together they demonstrate the myriad ways our bodies respond to our external environment.

Bears hibernate in winter, and if we live in a climate where the seasons change, we tend to slow down, too. In the days when many people farmed, that was a natural rhythm; people were less active in the winter. By the same token, construction workers get more exercise on the job in the warmer months.

So it may come as a surprise that the difference in physical activity from season to season is greater among people who are well educated and enjoy leisure pursuits than among manual laborers. It seems that if we have the option to be less active in the winter, we jump on it. Research worldwide shows a dip in physical activity in the colder months, by as much as 20 percent in a study of Michigan residents.

The bad news is that, for the most part, while we may be exercising less, we're eating just as much. The amount of weight gained by slacking off on exercise each winter—on average, a pound or two—can add up over the years.

Simply being aware of the likeliness of losing your mojo can help you keep it. When women participated in a lifestyle program that emphasized year-round fitness, they strapped on pedometers and reversed their usual winter

Burn More Fat in Winter

Here's a motivational fact: A study in Japan suggests we can make a greater change in body composition—that is, burn more fat—by doing the same amount of exercise in winter as we do in summer. Researchers believe this happens because our resting metabolism (basal metabolism) is higher in winter and more fatty acids are burned as fuel.

dip in activity. A review published in the *European Journal of Applied Psychology* concluded that simple steps could help, such as making people aware of opportunities to exercise indoors in winter. The same rules apply if it's July in Phoenix and the mercury just hit 120 degrees: Work out indoors, or if you must exercise outside, do it first thing in the morning or late in the day, when it's cooler.

Maximize Your Motivation

Some people get a kick from exercise. New research suggests that it's not endorphins that make us exercise-happy, but another group of molecules called endocannabinoids. If the name sounds familiar, it's probably because they bind to the same receptors in the brain as marijuana does for a feeling of pain-free well-being. Talk about a runner's high!

If you're not one of those people who get a rush from working out (there's new evidence that this may be genetic), here are some proven ways to encourage yourself. Up the ante by taking advantage of more than one.

Count your steps. In a study published in 2007 in the *Journal of the American Medical Association*, 2,767 study participants, mostly women, increased their steps by nearly 3,000 a day when they strapped on a pedometer.

Let the music take you. Listening to music increased the endurance of people exercising on a treadmill by 15 percent in a study published in 2008 in

EXERCISE AND YOUR MONTHLY CYCLE

In the old days, having your period was an ironclad excuse to get out of gym class. No more. Scientists have shown that there's no harm in exercising while you're menstruating. In fact, women are just as strong, just as fast then as at any other time of the month. "In terms of performance, the menstrual cycle doesn't have much impact, surprisingly," says Michael Deschenes, chairman of kinesiology and health sciences at the College of William and Mary in Williamsburg, Virginia.

Ann Caldwell Hooper, a PhD candidate at the University of New Mexico and lead researcher for a study published in a 2011 issue of the *Journal of Women's Health*, agrees, and adds an interesting finding that may explain why we were so eager to skip gym: When we exercise during our periods, we think we're working harder. Sometimes it even hurts. As part of the study, 189 women ran on the treadmill during various stages of their menstrual cycles, and rated their exertion levels at 65 percent of their max aerobic capacity. "We found that during the first 5 days of menstruation, performance doesn't change but perceived exertion and pain do," Hooper explains. "This might be tied to a lack of hormones, the very low estrogen and progesterone during menstruation. In other studies, estrogen has a damping effect on exercise pain." There was no difference in perceived exertion at any other time of the month.

What can we learn from this? Hooper and her team were trying to identify the optimal time to start an exercise program, which, as it turns out, is probably not the beginning of your cycle. Her advice: "Go easier on yourself if you're having your period and are uncomfortable. This is not the best time to push yourself or to evaluate the benefits of your fitness program."

Note: For women who take birth control pills, there was no difference in performance or perceived exertion across their cycles. So go ahead and exercise throughout your cycle, but if you're uncomfortable, cut yourself some slack. Brief sessions of strength training or stretching are often easier on these days than full-bore cardio.

Some yoga instructors advise students to avoid inversions during their periods because a shoulder stand or headstand reverses the downward flow of energy in the body during menstruation. Probably the best advice here is to know your own body; if inversions are uncomfortable or seem to affect your flow, it's better to skip them during this time.

the *Journal of Sport & Exercise Psychology*. Picking up the tempo of the songs you select will encourage you to pick up the pace of your aerobic exercise.

Make friends. People who exercised in a group quadrupled their exercise after 3 months, and were exercising even more than that after 9 months, according to a study in the *International Journal of Sport and Exercise Psychology*. (See Karen and Mary's story, opposite page.)

Be accountable. Participants who received regular phone calls (either automated or from a health educator) were exercising significantly more at the end of a year than those who didn't get the reminder phone call, according to a study at Stanford University that was published in 2007. Don't have a trainer who can call you? Ask a friend to do the deed; have him or her call every other week to ask how much you've worked out and congratulate you on your success.

Keep a log. Writing down how long you exercised can not only keep you working out, it can chart your progress—faster pace, longer endurance, bigger weights. Use the log sheet starting on page 343.

Get a dog. If you've been trying to convince your partner to get a pet, here's a new argument. A number of studies point to the fitness benefits for dog owners. A study in Australia published in 2008 found that people who adopted dogs increased their exercise time by 400 percent, as compared with those in a control group who didn't get the pets.

Short on time? Do what you can. Research shows that accomplishing your workout in segments as brief as 10 minutes can be just as good as a single session.

Still Need Motivation?

Physical activity isn't just a "wonder drug"—it's one of the pillars of your circadian rhythm program. Craft an exercise routine that works with, not against, your internal rhythm and it will help reinforce the elements of healthy living that you've set up for yourself.

But if you're one of those people who just don't enjoy working out, don't despair. Let's work on boosting your motivation by discovering the many wonderful things that exercise can do for you. And be sure to reread this section anytime you feel that your motivation is starting to sag.

THE BUDDY SYSTEM: WALKING TOGETHER KEPT KAREN AND MARY ON TRACK

Test panelists Karen Posten and Mary Davis joined the Belly Melt Diet program together, so they decided to do their morning walks together as well. Doing so not only sped up their weight loss but also gave the friends cherished time together. "We have a rabbit who waits for us," Mary says. "On the way home, there's a tree with blossoms that have fallen to create a carpet of red." The two also signed up for a bird calling class so they could recognize the birds they hear singing early every morning.

As Mary and Karen walked, they'd share tips for sticking with the BMD plan. "Mary travels for her job, and she told me how she keeps healthy snacks in the car, where they'll be handy," Karen says. She adds, "Walking together has become a wonderful habit for us. We talk over our day and our struggles with busyness. Mary's support has been invaluable in my sticking with the program."

Why exercise? To live longer. Let's start with the biggest benefit of all: Exercise can add years to your life. The equation is that simple—more exercise, more healthy, longer life. Physical activity can extend your life in two ways. First, it reduces the risk of a variety of diseases, from diabetes to the common cold. Just as important, it also works on the microscopic level, literally keeping your cells vibrant and young.

When you jog or take a bike ride, or perform a series of weight-lifting exercises, you're toning your body on the inside as well as the outside, making your organs resistant to the ravages of disease. The benefits come quickly. In some of the studies we'll look at, reverses in risk factors for disease occurred after just 12 weeks of regular exercise.

Your heart works harder when you exercise. But, you may ask, wouldn't that make it wear out sooner? Sounds logical, doesn't it? But speeding up your heart rate and then returning to a normal pulse makes your heart more efficient. Sure, it works harder when you exercise, but once you're fit, it will beat at a slower rate all day. Work hard for 1 hour, then cruise for the other 23: That's a formula for good health. In fact, scientists reviewing the literature for an article in a 2010 issue of the *Journal of Obesity* concluded that "cardiorespiratory fitness is a more powerful predictor of cardiovascular and mortality risk than body weight."

Keeping your heart fit through exercise can keep it beating longer, lengthening your life. In a recent study at Harvard Medical School, researchers found that the fittest among the nearly 3,000 participants reduced their risk of dying from heart disease almost ninefold over 20 years. That's because regular exercise reduces risk factors for heart disease, including high cholesterol, inflammation agents, and high blood pressure. In another study, published in *Medicine & Science in Sports & Exercise,* sedentary adults were assigned to a 12-week exercise program that combined aerobics and strength training. Not only did the subjects increase their aerobic capacity by 10 percent and their strength by a whopping 38 percent, but they also lowered the levels of

C-reactive protein in their blood, an important marker for heart disease. Other studies show significant improvements in cholesterol after a regimen of exercise. Women who began a 16-week weight-training program lowered their LDL cholesterol by almost 18 percent and their triglycerides by 28 percent. A study at Arizona State University found that women who were physically active had fewer risk factors for both cardiovascular disease and type 2 diabetes. Bonus points: They had smaller waists, less body fat, and lower BMIs.

On the flip side, researchers at Ochsner Health System in Baton Rouge, Louisiana, have bad news for couch potatoes. They examined the physical activity and health of 120,000 people and found that women who sat for 6 hours a day raised their risk of dying during the 14 years of the study by 37 percent, as compared with women who sat fewer than 3 hours a day.

Need more encouragement to get off your duff? There's plenty. Exercise has been shown to decrease the risk of a number of cancers. Women who exercise regularly cut their risk of endometrial cancer by 30 percent, breast cancer by 25 percent, and ovarian cancer by 20 percent. Other studies point to risk reductions for lung cancer as well as colorectal and other gastric cancers. Exercise can even help people who have already been diagnosed. In a study of 3,000 women with hormone-responsive breast cancer tumors, walking 3 to 5 hours a week halved their risk of dying over 10 years.

You know that exercise burns glucose. It also helps your body manage blood glucose better, resulting in lower levels. Because it allows your body to metabolize blood sugar efficiently, exercise can ward off type 2 diabetes and help these patients regulate blood sugar with less medication or even none at all. People with type 1 diabetes, who take insulin, may be able to manage their blood sugar with less insulin.

Now let's talk about the other way that exercise keeps you young—by keeping your cells fit and trim, too. A key measure of the aging process is the length of our chromosomes. As we get older, our chromosomes literally shrink, leading to disruptions in the function of our cells. Chromosomes are protected by telomeres, which sit out on the end like aglets on the ends of your shoelaces (yes, those plastic tips have a name!). Wear your telomeres down and things start falling apart.

Research has shown that exercising regularly reduces telomere shrinkage, which makes working out one of the few proven antiaging activities. Scientists aren't sure how this happens, but they theorize that aerobic exercise may increase the activity of the enzyme telomerase, which repairs telomeres, or it may increase the production of proteins that stabilize the telomeres. Another possibility is that exercise protects telomeres by making cells more resistant to stress. While you're exercising, it stresses your cells. Sounds bad, but in the long run, it's good. That's because exercise trains your cells to better handle the burden of removing the by-products of glucose metabolism throughout the day. Exercise gooses your system to become more efficient at cleansing your body of toxic wastes like free radicals, or excess ions shed in the metabolism of glucose, which can damage cells. A healthy cell is less vulnerable to disease. In a recent experiment at McMaster University in Hamilton, Ontario, mice that exercised in the study moderated or eliminated almost every effect of aging; they didn't even go gray.

Exercise can even help guard against the ravages of Alzheimer's. "Physical inactivity is one of the most prominent risk factors for dementia," according to a study published in the *Journal of Alzheimer's Disease.* How exercise protects our brains isn't fully understood, although we do know that it keeps the brain healthy by enhancing cell mechanisms that repair oxidative damage (disarming the free radicals we talked about earlier) and improving cardiovascular function and metabolism within brain cells.

Why exercise? To build better bones. The sad truth is, our bones peak much sooner than we do. They're at their strongest in our late twenties or early thirties. After that, it's pretty much all downhill, though some of us slide a lot faster than others. Estrogen helps us make strong bones; when that hormone takes a powder at menopause, our bones can suffer big-time, leading to osteopenia (thinning bones) or full-blown osteoporosis, with a much higher fracture risk. One of the most important things we can do to preserve our bones, whether we're 26 and still building them or 56 and trying to hang on to what we've got, is to exercise. Strength training, using barbells, free weights, weight machines, or elastic bands, puts pressure on the bones—that's why it's also called resistance training. Working against resistance prompts our bones to stay strong. High-intensity training—using heavier weights that work your muscles to fatigue in fewer reps—is most effective. In one study, women with osteoporosis increased bone density in their spines by 2.8 percent in just 5 months of strength training.

Why exercise? To get smarter. Walking can make your brain bigger. No fooling. In a recent study published in the *Proceedings of the National Academy of Science,* researchers asked 120 sedentary adults to walk three times a week, working up to 40 minutes each time, or do a less aerobic activity like yoga. Since the average age of the subjects was mid-sixties, a time when the brain is shrinking, it was no surprise that after a year the second group lost 1.4 percent volume of the hippocampus, the seat of memory and the all-important SCN (this was actually less than the researchers had anticipated—scary, huh?). Meanwhile, the walking group had a 2 percent increase in hippocampus volume.

That's just one among many studies that prove the value of exercise in improving cognitive function. People who exercise also perform better on tests that measure problem solving, attention, reasoning, and long-term memory. In his book, *Brain Rules,* John Medina, PhD, recommends aerobic activity augmented by a strength-training regimen for even greater benefits.

It makes sense that exercise would strengthen the mind. Your brain consumes 20 percent of the caloric energy used by your body, so keeping the cardiovascular system in tip-top shape means that your brain is getting the glucose and oxygen it needs.

Why exercise? To feel better day in, day out. Exercise is one of the most potent mood lifters there is. Studies since the 1970s have shown that physically active people are less likely to be depressed than their physically inactive counterparts. In a landmark 1999 study on depression at Duke University, participants experienced as much improvement in their moods by doing aerobic exercise as by taking antidepressants. A follow-up study in 2007 yielded similar results. Scientists theorize that exercise keeps us on an even keel by regulating the brain chemicals norepinephrine and serotonin.

Keeping physically active can even blunt the assault of our nemesis, the common cold. A study published in the *British Journal of Sports Medicine* in 2010 followed 1,002 adults for 12 weeks during fall and winter. Those who did aerobic exercise 5 or more days a week suffered upper-respiratory-tract infections on 43 percent fewer days than those who didn't work out regularly. Likewise, the exercisers saw a 40 percent reduction in the severity of symptoms.

Why exercise? To help drop those pesky pounds. The math is simple: To lose 1 pound of fat, you need to burn 3,500 calories. You can burn 500 calories an hour in a variety of ways—running, swimming laps, playing tennis, or working out on a treadmill at the gym. Exercise at a vigorous pace an hour a day for a week and you've burned the equivalent of a pound of fat. That's the reason those *Biggest Loser* contestants hit the gym every day. Exercise, coupled with a healthy eating plan, can melt pounds away. The National Weight Control Registry keeps track of people who've been able to maintain a significant weight loss—the ones who are successful where so many of us fail. Registry members have lost an average of 66 pounds and kept it off for an average of 5.5 years. What's their secret? A whopping 94 percent exercise regularly—mostly walking—to help maintain their weight loss. Another large-scale study confirms it. Looking at the exercise patterns and the weight of women in the Harvard Nurses' Health Study from 1989 to 2005, researchers discovered that those who exercised 30 minutes a day maintained their weight or even lost a few pounds, while others who worked out fewer than 15 minutes a day gained more than 4 pounds on average over those 16 years.

Beyond the fundamentals of thermodynamics, exercise can help boost your weight-loss plan in a variety of ways. First and foremost, it changes the composition of your body, building lean muscle while eliminating fat. Not only does this result in a healthier, more attractive shape, but it creates a body that burns more calories per pound, day after day. A pound of muscle burns 6 or 7 calories a day (this is your "resting metabolism," the number of calories your body needs to pump blood, digest food, and accomplish all the other internal activities of daily life). On the other hand, fat, essentially a storage mechanism, burns few or no calories. That pound of muscle is busy burning those calories all day, every day.

Experts tell us that exercise does other things, too, to help us maintain a healthy body weight. In an analysis of weight-loss studies spanning several decades, Danish researchers in 2010 concluded that exercise can help your body regulate its weight at the cellular level by stimulating enzymes and making cells more sensitive to hormones like insulin. In addition, exercise keeps our body's transportation network, the cardiovascular system, in good shape for moving nutrients into our cells and flushing out waste products. Finally, by blunting the effects of stress, exercise can help us battle stress-induced snacking.

My Belly Melt

"I never feel hungry!"

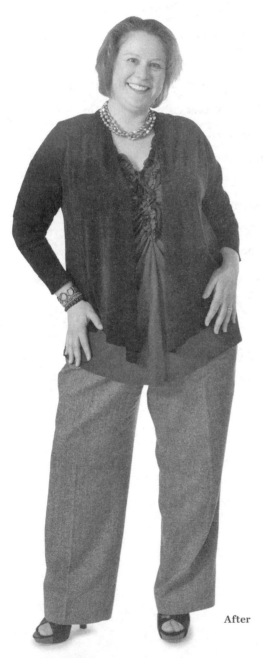

After

Tracy Hausknecht

AGE: 38

POUNDS LOST: 13.8 in 35 days

POUNDS LOST IN 3-DAY RESET: 6

ALLOVER INCHES LOST: 16.75

INCHES FROM WAIST LOST: 3

BODY FAT LOST: 3.1 percent

Tracy Hausknecht was off to a jackrabbit start, dropping 6 pounds in Phase 1 of the BMD plan. By the end of 5 weeks, she had more than doubled that loss and reduced her measurements by a whopping 16¾ inches. Her friends have noticed her sleeker physique. Her husband asked her if she was going to keep going, and she told him she would because the program was so easy to follow and because it had made the family's diet healthier.

Success Story

Tracy has always been an athlete, but in recent years the busy life of an active mom packed on extra pounds. "I'm constantly running with the kids. I'd eat their leftover cookies, grab some chips," she says. "I was always foraging for the wrong kind of food." When the opportunity came to test-drive the BMD program, she jumped at it. She likes the multifaceted plan, with suggestions for better sleep, diet, and exercise. "All the pieces work together; it feels organic."

BMD has reinvented Tracy as a morning person, someone who wakes up more easily and slips into a good morning routine. "I have no problem falling asleep. As soon as my head hits the pillow, I'm gone," but getting up was another matter entirely. With the plan, she set a standard wake-up time of 6:30. "For years, I tried to get up at 6:00, but I've discovered that 6:30 is my circadian rhythm, and I have to

Before

work with that. I drink a glass of water, walk the dog for 20 minutes, get my middle schooler on the bus, hit Facebook for a few minutes, get the little one up, jump in the shower, put my 9-year-old on the bus, and head for work at 8:20, where I'll eat breakfast at my desk." Everything has fallen into place. "This program changed my wake-up rhythm for the better.

"My problem was never cravings; it was that I ate whatever was available," Tracy continues. "Now healthy eating is part of my routine." She makes sure that she always has the right food on hand, packing berries to nibble on at soccer practice and turkey roll-ups with spinach that she can eat in the car at Girl Scouts or a soccer game.

Tracy loves her Pilates routine, so she did that for her afternoon strength training. "I just did a standing split on the Reformer," she brags with a big smile. "I couldn't do that 5 weeks ago."

Only one thing disappoints: that her "after" shot was taken at 5 weeks. "Just wait until you see me in another 5!" she says.

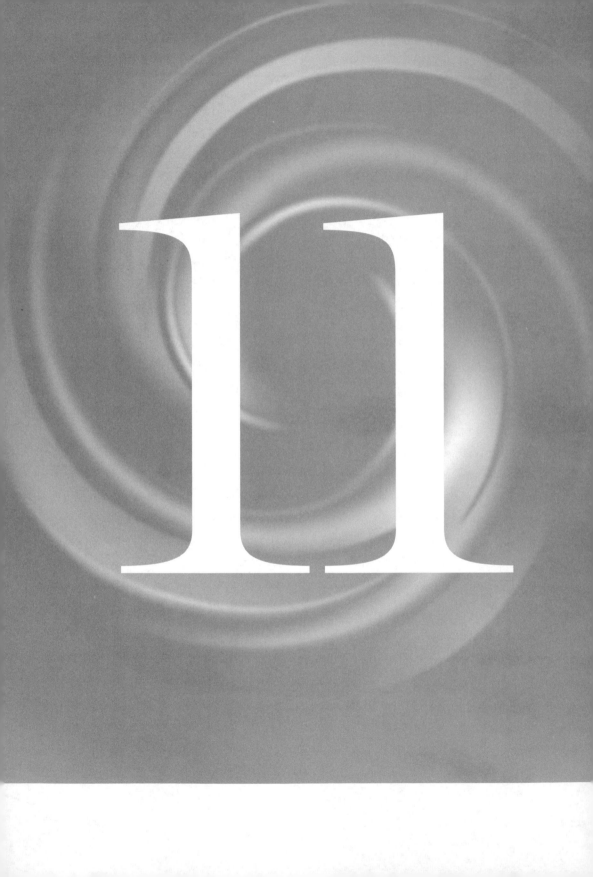

The Belly Melt Diet Workouts

We'll make this as easy as possible: Get out there and walk, preferably in the morning (for a refresher on why, see page 250). In the beginning, especially if you haven't been active for a while, simply lace up your shoes and head out for at least 20 minutes. As for effort, imagine a level that registers a 6, 7, or 8 on a scale of 1 to 10. As you continue your workouts, you'll notice that you can move faster for the same amount of effort; this means your body is becoming more efficient.

If you're up for something a bit more involved or want to try something else, here are 20-minute interval workouts created by *Prevention* magazine's fitness expert Wayne Westcott, PhD, exercise science research director, Quincy College in Quincy, Massachusetts, and his associate, Rita La Rosa Loud, exercise science instructor, Quincy College. Again, you'll see just how simple these workouts are. Interval training increased fat burn by an astounding 36 percent for subjects in a study at the University of Ontario. You'll not only burn more fat but also, like many people, find that breaking your exercise into segments makes it seem to go by much faster.

Burn the Fat

EFFORT LEVELS SCALE				
1	2	3	4	5
Low Effort	Low to Moderate Effort	Moderate Effort	Moderate to High Effort	High Effort

Treadmill/Walking/Rowing Machine (easy)

3 min. Warmup/Level 1

15 min. Level 3 (slight hills)

3 min. Cooldown/Level 1

Stationary Bike

3 min. Warmup/Level 1

3 min. Level 2

3 min. Level 3

3 min. Level 4

3 min. Level 3

3 min. Level 2

3 min. Cooldown/Level 1

Treadmill/Walking/Rowing Machine (moderate)*

3 min. Warmup/Level 1

2 min. Level 3

2 min. Level 4

2 min. Level 3

2 min. Level 4

2 min. Level 3

2 min. Level 4

2 min. Level 3

3 min. Cooldown/Level 1

(*If you master this, break into 3-minute alternating intervals.)

We've set up your workout so that you do a little each day, which will keep you on a regular workout "cycle" but also keep your workouts from taking over your life. Feel free to switch it up to fit your own rhythm; just try to do them in the afternoon (for maximum effect) and at least twice a week, with a day of rest in between (it's during the resting phase that muscles recover and get leaner). We've given you two options—workouts that use your body weight, and dumbbells—so you can do what works best with your body, budget, and schedule. Also, feel free to rotate the workouts, to keep them fresh and to keep you from getting bored. If you like what you see or you feel the exercises getting easier, try the Challenge Yourself option for each move, or turn to page 298 for an advanced workout. Remember to finish your workout with the easy stretch moves (the same for whatever workout you choose). Stretching after strength training maximizes results!

UPPER-BODY WORKOUT

(Mondays and Thursdays) Descriptions of your upper-body exercises begin on page 273.

Body Weight Workout

THE EXERCISES: Pushup, Chair Pullup, Bench Dip

THE STRETCHES: Doorway Inside Stretch, Doorway Outside Stretch

Dumbbell Workout

THE EXERCISES: Bench Press, Bent Row, Standing Press, Standing Curl, Lying Triceps Extension

THE STRETCHES: Doorway Inside Stretch, Doorway Outside Stretch

LOWER-BODY WORKOUT

(Tuesdays and Fridays) Descriptions of your lower-body exercises begin on page 283.

Body Weight Workout

THE EXERCISES: Squat, Side Lunge, Heel Raise, Trunk Curl, Trunk Extension

THE STRETCHES: Figure 4 Stretch, Standing Bent-Knee Stretch, Letter T Stretch

Dumbbell Workout

THE EXERCISES: Dumbbell Squat, Dumbbell Side Lunge, Dumbbell Heel Raise, Trunk Curl, Trunk Extension

THE STRETCHES: Figure 4 Stretch, Standing Bent-Knee Stretch, Letter T Stretch

THE BIG 4 FLAT-BELLY MOVES

(Add to workouts above or do on other days, twice a week.) Descriptions of your Big 4 Flat-Belly Moves begin on page 294.

Build Lean, Sleek Muscle

It's a simple plan—15 to 20 minutes of strength training and stretching four times a week. In a study published in the *Physician and Sportsmedicine,* 1,600 adults (mostly women) averaged a 3.1-pound muscle gain and 3.7-pound loss of body fat after just 10 weeks of strength training. And a study at the University of Michigan found that adults who strength-trained for 18 to 20 weeks added an average of 2.42 pounds of lean muscle and increased their strength by 25 to 30 percent. Be sure to slot in your strength workouts in the late afternoon and early evening, when, as we've learned, they're most efficient (see page 251 for more details).

Pushup

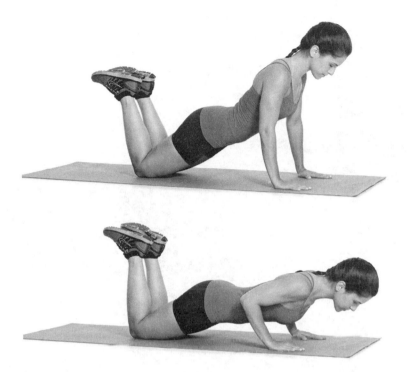

Targets:
Chest, front shoulders, rear arms
(pectoralis major, anterior deltoids,
triceps)

Do the move:
Assume a modified plank position, with
your feet together, legs bent, knees on
the floor, hands on the floor slightly
wider than shoulder-width apart, arms
straight. Slowly lower your body until
your upper arms are nearly horizontal,
then slowly return to starting position.
Inhale when you lower your body, exhale
when you raise it.

How many?
Do two sets of 10 repetitions.

Challenge yourself:
Try full-plank pushups, with your legs
straight and knees off the floor. Full or
modified, work up to three sets of
20 repetitions.

Chair Pullup

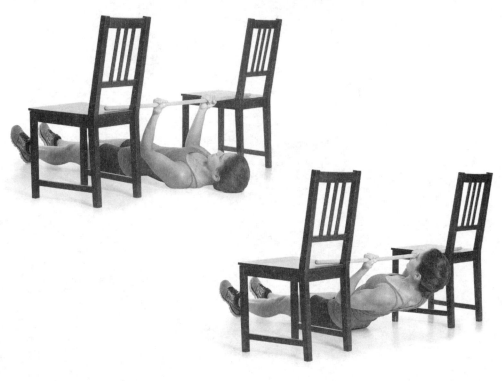

Targets:
Upper back, rear shoulders, front arms, lower back (latissimus dorsi, posterior deltoids, biceps, erector spinae)

Do the move:
Place a sturdy broom handle across two chair seats about 2 feet apart. Lie face-up on the floor with your chest under the broom handle. Grasp the broom handle with an underhand grip and slowly pull your body up until your chest almost touches the handle, then slowly lower back to the floor. Exhale as you rise; inhale as you lower down. Keep your body straight and your heels on the floor throughout the exercise.

How many?
Do two sets of 5 repetitions.

Challenge yourself:
Work up to 10 repetitions, then up to three sets of 10.

Bench Dip

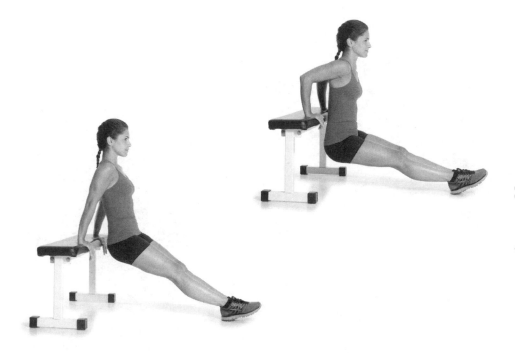

Targets:

Rear arms, chest, front shoulders (triceps, pectoralis major, anterior deltoids)

Do the move:

Sit on the edge of a flat chair or bench with your palms on the front edge, legs straight to the front, heels on the floor. Lift your hips upward by extending your arms, keeping your hips just far enough forward to clear the chair seat. Slowly lower your hips down until your elbows are flexed about 90 degrees. Then slowly press back up to the starting position. Inhale as you lower your body; exhale as you raise it. Keep your back and legs straight throughout.

How many?

Do two sets of 10 repetitions.

Challenge yourself:

Work up to 20 repetitions, then three sets of 20.

Dumbbell Bench Press

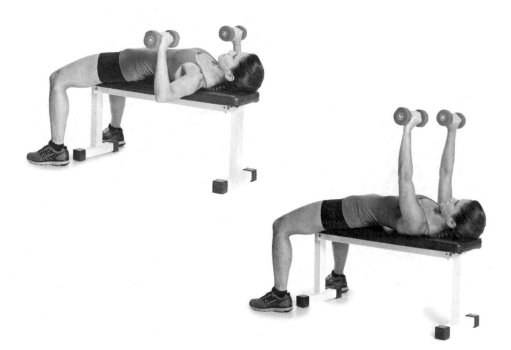

Targets:
Chest, front shoulders, rear arms (pectoralis major, anterior deltoids, triceps)

Do the move:
Lie face-up on a flat bench with your elbows flexed away from your body and directly below the wrists with a 7-pound dumbbell in each hand lightly touching your chest. Slowly press both dumbbells upward until your arms are fully extended, then slowly return to the starting position. Exhale as you raise the dumbbells, and inhale as you lower them. Keep your head and hips on the bench, and your feet on the floor for stability.

How many?
Do two sets of 10 repetitions.

Challenge yourself:
Work up to 15 repetitions, then three sets of 15.

Dumbbell Bent Row

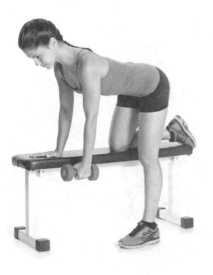

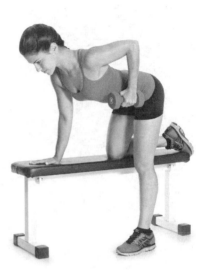

Targets:

Upper back, rear shoulders, front arms (latissimus dorsi, posterior deltoids, biceps)

Do the move:

Place your right hand and right knee on a flat bench, back approximately horizontal, a 7-pound dumbbell in left hand, left arm straight. Slowly pull the dumbbell upward until it lightly touches your chest on the left side. Pause, then slowly lower the dumbbell to the starting position for 10 repetitions. Change position and repeat with your right arm.

How many?

Do two sets of 10 repetitions.

Challenge yourself:

Work up to 15 repetitions, then three sets of 15.

Dumbbell Standing Press

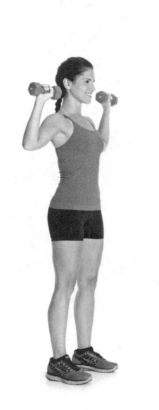
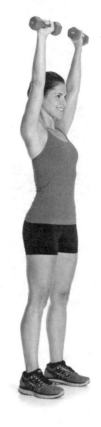

Targets:
Shoulders, rear arms (deltoids, triceps)

Do the move:
Stand tall with your feet shoulder-width apart, a 5-pound dumbbell in each hand lightly touching your shoulders. Slowly press both hands upward until your arms are fully extended, then slowly return to the starting position. Exhale as you extend up; inhale as you return to your shoulders. Keep your back straight and resist the temptation to bend backwards or sideways.

How many?
Do two sets of 10 repetitions.

Challenge yourself:
Work up to 15 repetitions.

Dumbbell Standing Curl

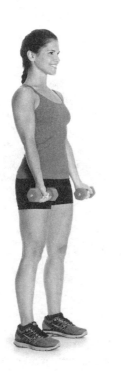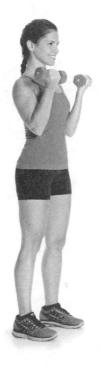

Targets:
Front arms (biceps)

Do the move:
Stand tall with your feet shoulder-width apart and a 5-pound dumbbell in each hand, arms hanging straight down. Slowly curl both dumbbells upward until your elbows are fully flexed. Pause and slowly lower the dumbbells to the starting position. Exhale as you raise the dumbbells; inhale as you lower them. Keep your back straight and your upper arms vertical against your sides throughout the exercise. Resist the temptation to bend backward.

How many?
Do two sets of 10 repetitions.

Challenge yourself:
Work up to 15 repetitions.

Dumbbell Lying Triceps Extension

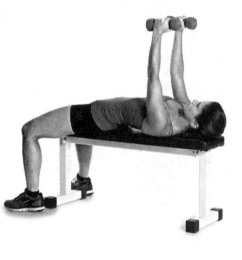

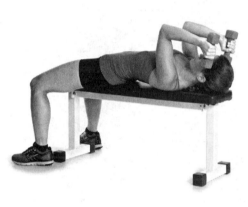

Targets:
Rear arms (triceps)

Do the move:
Lie face-up on a flat bench with your arms extended upward, a 3-pound dumbbell in each hand. Without moving your upper arms, slowly lower the dumbbells by bending your elbows until the dumbbells are next to your ears. Pause and slowly lift them to the starting position. Inhale as you lower the dumbbells; exhale as you raise them. Keep your feet on the floor for stability, and your head and hips securely on the bench. Your upper arms should be vertical and stationary throughout.

How many?
Do two sets of 10 repetitions.

Challenge yourself:
Work up to 15 repetitions.

Doorway Inside Stretch

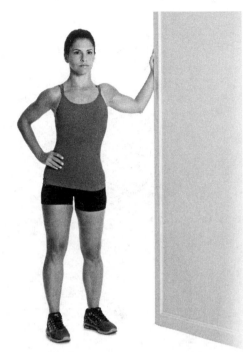

Targets:
Front shoulders, front arms (anterior deltoids, biceps)

Do the move:
Stand tall in a doorway, feet shoulder-width apart, with your left hand on the inside of the left side of the door frame at shoulder level. Turn your upper body to the right until your left front shoulder and left front arm are comfortably stretched, and hold that position for 20 seconds. Repeat the stretch on the other side, using your right hand and the right side of the door frame. Breathe normally throughout.

How many?
Do two 20-second stretches on each side.

Challenge yourself:
As your muscles become accustomed to being stretched, you can hold the second repetition in a slightly greater stretched position. Work up to 30-second stretches.

Doorway Outside Stretch

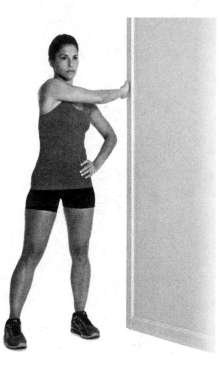

Targets:
Rear shoulders, rear arms (posterior deltoids, triceps)

Do the move:
Stand tall in a doorway, feet shoulder-width apart, with your right hand on the outside of the left side of the door frame at shoulder height. Turn your upper body to the right until your right rear shoulder and right rear arm are comfortably stretched, and hold that position for 20 seconds. Repeat the stretch on the other side, using your left hand and the right side of the door frame. Breathe normally throughout.

How many?
Do two 20-second stretches on each side.

Challenge yourself:
As your muscles become accustomed to being stretched, you can hold the second repetition in a slightly greater stretched position. Work up to 30-second stretches.

Squat

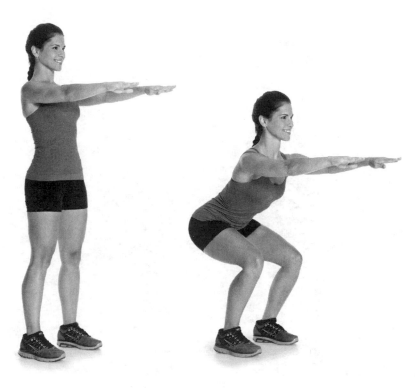

Targets:
Front and rear thighs, buttocks (quadriceps, hamstrings, gluteals)

Do the move:
Stand tall, feet shoulder-width apart or slightly wider, with arms extended at shoulder height. Slowly lower your hips down and back until your thighs are horizontal, then slowly return to standing position by extending your knees and hips. Inhale on the downward movement; exhale as you rise. Keep your head up, your back straight, and your knees directly above your feet throughout.

How many?
Do two sets of 10 repetitions.

Challenge yourself:
Add repetitions, up to 20, or do three sets.

Side Lunge

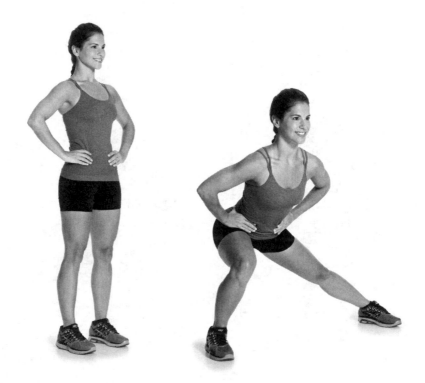

Targets:
Inner and outer thighs (hip adductors and hip abductors)

Do the move:
Stand tall with your feet shoulder-width apart and hands on your hips. Take a big step to the left with your left foot while lowering your hips down and back until your right thigh is nearly horizontal. Return to starting position. Inhale when you're moving down; exhale when you're moving up. Keep your head up, your back straight, and the knee of your stationary leg directly above your foot.

How many?
After 10 repetitions with your left foot, repeat the exercise with your right foot moving to the right. Do two sets.

Challenge yourself:
Increase repetitions to 20, then increase the number of sets to three.

Heel Raise

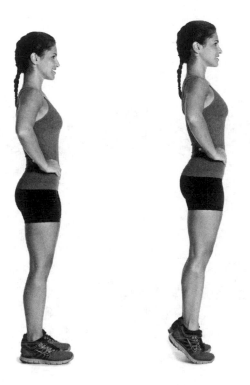

Targets:

Calves (gastrocnemius, soleus)

Do the move:

Stand with your feet slightly less than shoulder-width apart, hands on your hips. Slowly lift both heels off the floor as far as you can. Pause, then slowly return heels to the floor. Exhale during the upward movement; inhale as you move down. Keep your head up, and your back and legs straight.

How many?

Do two sets of 10 repetitions.

Challenge yourself:

Increase repetitions. When you can do 15 comfortably, add a third set.

Trunk Extension

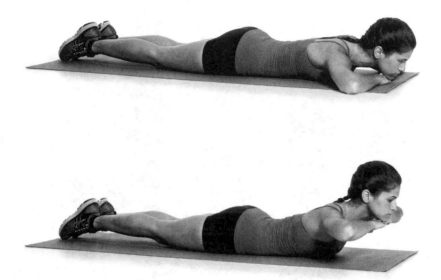

Targets:
Lower back (erector spinae)

Do the move:
Lie face-down on the floor with your
hands clasped loosely under your chin.
Slowly lift your chest off the floor until
your back muscles are fully contracted.
Pause, then slowly return to the starting
position. Exhale as you raise your chest;
inhale as you lower it. Maintain a neutral
head position throughout.

How many?
Do two sets of 10 repetitions.

Challenge yourself:
Increase repetitions. When you can do
15 comfortably, add a third set.

Dumbbell Squat

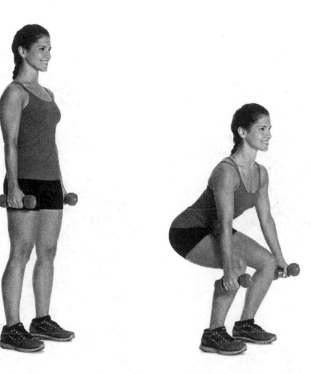

Targets:
Front and rear thighs, buttocks (quadri-ceps, hamstrings, gluteals)

Do the move:
Follow the instructions for the Squat (page 283), holding a 10-pound dumbbell in each hand, with your arms straight down.

How many?
Do three sets of 10 repetitions.

Challenge yourself:
Increase repetitions. When you can comfortably do 15, graduate to heavier dumbbells.

Dumbbell Side Lunge

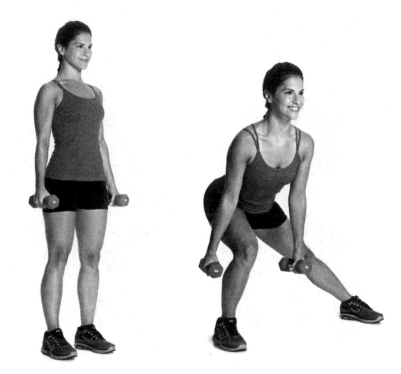

Targets:

Inner and outer thighs (hip adductors and hip abductors)

Do the move:

Follow the instructions for the Side Lunge (page 284), holding a 5-pound dumbbell in each hand at waist level.

How many?

Do two sets of 10 repetitions, the same as for the Side Lunge.

Challenge yourself:

Increase repetitions. When you can complete 15 comfortably, graduate to the next heavier weight.

Dumbbell Heel Raise

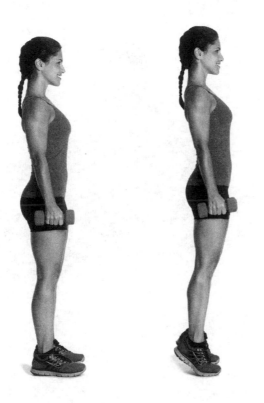

Targets:
Calves (gastrocnemius, soleus)

Do the move:
Follow the instructions for the Heel Raise (page 285), holding a 10-pound dumbbell in each hand, with arms hanging straight down.

How many?
Do two sets of 10 repetitions.

Challenge yourself:
Increase repetitions. When you can do 15 comfortably, graduate to the next heavier set of dumbbells.

Figure 4 Stretch

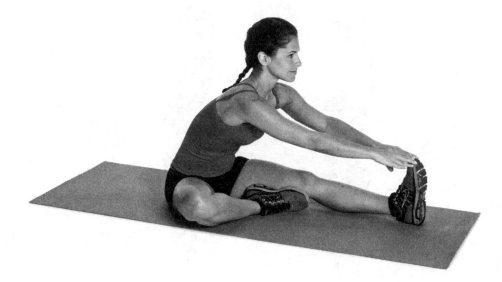

Targets:
Rear thighs, lower back, upper back
(hamstrings, erector spinae, latissimus
dorsi)

Do the move:
Sit on the floor with your left leg
straight out in front of you and your
right leg bent so that your right foot
rests against your left inner thigh.
Reach forward as far as comfortable
and grasp your left leg, ankle, or foot
with your hands. Hold the stretch for
20 seconds. Repeat the stretch,
reversing sides. Breathe normally
throughout the stretch.

How many?
Do two 20-second stretches on each side.

Challenge yourself:
As your muscles become accustomed
to being stretched, you will be able to
hold a greater stretch on the second
repetition. You can increase each
stretch to 30 seconds.

Standing Bent-Knee Stretch

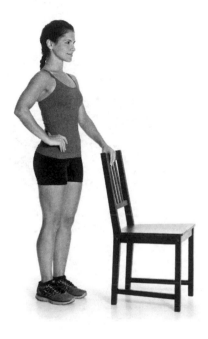

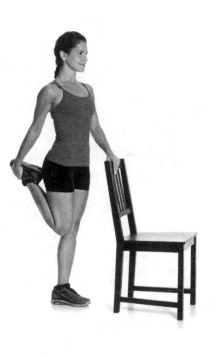

Targets:

Front thighs, hips (quadriceps, iliacus, psoas)

Do the move:

Standing tall on your left leg with your left hand on a chair back for stability, bend your right knee and grasp your right foot with your right hand. Move your hips forward until you feel the stretch in your right thigh. Hold the stretch for 20 seconds, then repeat on the other side. Breathe normally throughout.

How many?

Do two 20-second stretches on each side.

Challenge yourself:

As your muscles become accustomed to being stretched, you will be able to hold a greater stretch on the second repetition. You can increase each stretch to 30 seconds.

Letter T Stretch

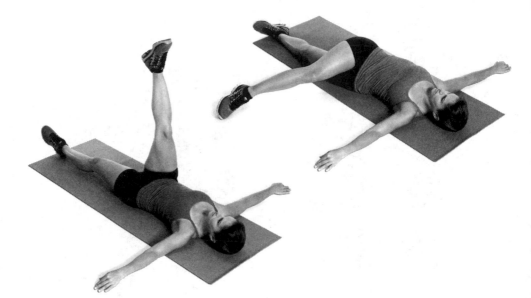

Targets:
Lower back, rear thighs, buttocks, side midsection (erector spinae, hamstrings, gluteals, obliques)

Do the move:
Lie face-up on the floor with your legs straight and arms extended to form a T. Lift your right leg straight up, then across your body, bringing your foot as close as you can to your left hand. Hold the stretch for 20 seconds, then return to the starting position. Repeat on the other side. Breathe normally throughout the stretch.

How many?
Do two 20-second stretches on each side.

Challenge yourself:
As your muscles become accustomed to being stretched, you will be able to hold a greater stretch on the second repetition. You can increase each stretch to 30 seconds.

5-Minute Belly Buster:
The Big 4 Flat-Belly Moves

When researchers at San Diego State tested the best ab exercises, these moves ranked highest—so you know you're getting the most belly busting for your buck. This supercharged workout reinvents the classic crunch. "I've used this routine for 30 years with great results. It's a very safe way to get a hard workout," says workout creator Wayne Westcott, PhD.

The first three exercises are sequenced to fatigue the fast-twitch fibers in your muscles, and the final exercise digs deeper to your harder-to-fatigue slow-twitch fibers. "The key is not taking breaks when you do this workout, so you don't give your fast-twitch muscles time to recover," Dr. Westcott says.

Beginners should try twice a week; more advanced exercisers can up the ante to four times (particularly during beach season!). Do the moves slowly and deliberately, with as little transition time as possible between exercises.

1
Trunk Curl

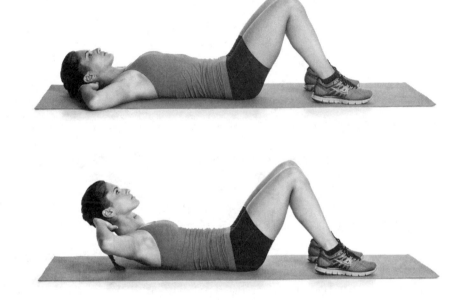

Targets:

Front midsection (rectus abdominis)

Do the move:

Lie face-up on the floor with your knees bent, feet on the floor, and your hands clasped loosely behind your head. Slowly curl your upper back off the floor until your lower back is pressed firmly against the floor. Pause, then slowly return to the starting position. Exhale as you rise; inhale as you lower back down. Keep your head position neutral throughout.

How many?

Do a set of 10 repetitions, then proceed immediately to #2.

2

Single-Knee Trunk Curl

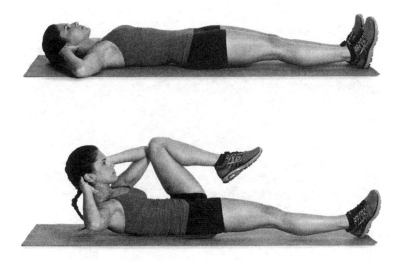

Targets:
Front midsection (rectus abdominis, rectus femoris, iliacus, psoas)

Do the move:
Lie face-up on the floor with your legs straight and your hands clasped loosely behind your head. Slowly curl your upper back off the floor until your lower back is pressed firmly against the floor. As you curl up, bring your left knee back to touch your left elbow. Slowly lower your upper back to the floor, extending your left leg back to the legs-straight position at the same time. For the second curl, repeat the move, touching your right elbow to your right knee. Exhale as you lift your trunk; inhale as you lower it. Keep your head position neutral throughout.

How many?
Do a set of 10 repetitions, alternating legs for each rep, then proceed immediately to #3.

3

Double-Knee Trunk Curl

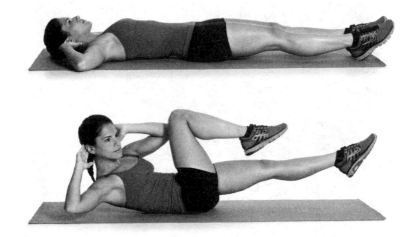

Targets:

Front midsection, side midsection (rectus abdominis, external obliques, internal obliques, rectus femoris, iliacus, psoas)

Do the move:

Lie face-up on the floor with your legs straight and your hands clasped loosely behind your head. Slowly curl your upper back off the floor until your lower back is pressed firmly against the floor. Maintaining that position, lift both legs 6 inches off the floor. Keeping your left leg straight, bring your right leg back and turn your torso to the right, touching your left elbow to your right knee. As you return your right leg to the starting position, repeat the motion on the other side, bringing your left leg back and turning your torso to the left, touching your right elbow to your left knee. Maintain a neutral head position, and don't hold your breath.

How many?

Do a set of 10 repetitions, alternating sides for each rep, then proceed immediately to #4.

4

Legs-Up Trunk Curl

Targets:

Front midsection (rectus abdominis, rectus femoris, iliacus, psoas)

Do the move:

Lie face-up on the floor with your legs straight and your hands clasped loosely behind your head. Raise both legs upward, as close to vertical as possible; you'll maintain this position throughout the exercise. Slowly curl your upper back off the floor, then slowly lower to the starting position. Exhale as you rise; inhale as you lower your trunk, and maintain a neutral head position. (If you want more of a challenge, touch your elbows to your knees.)

How many?

Do one set of 10 repetitions. Congratulations! You're done—and four moves closer to the flat belly of your dreams.

The Super-Lean Workout

Whether you've mastered the previous workouts or you're looking for something new, these multitasking exercises will supercharge your workout. For best results, do them once or twice a week instead of your strength-training routine or add a move or two if you like certain exercises.

Before you know it, you'll see even more results: firmer muscles, a leaner body, and you'll feel great, too.

Hip, Hip Away

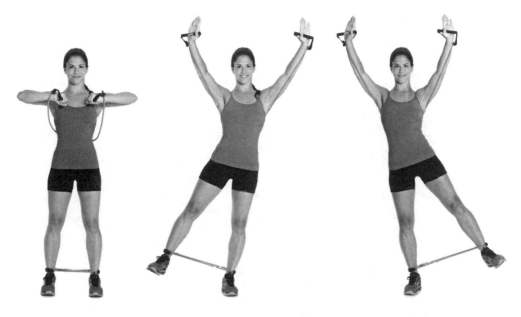

Targets:
Hips, butt, outer thighs, shoulders (gluteals, abductors, deltoids)

Do the move:
Stand tall with your feet hip-width apart, with a taut resistant band (without handles) tied around your ankles. Place a second resistance band around your mid-upper back and under your arms, holding a handle in each hand and arms at shoulder level, with your elbows bent 90 degrees. As you slowly press your right leg out to the side, raise your arms overhead, keeping your wrists in line with your forearms. Return to starting position, and repeat exercise with the left leg. Inhale as you bring your arms down; exhale as you raise them. Keep toes, knees, hips, and shoulders facing forward, and maintain a straight back and contracted abdominals throughout.

How many?
Start with two sets of 10 repetitions each; work up to three sets of 15.

Challenge yourself:
When you can do 15 repetitions comfortably, graduate to the next heavier-resistance band.

Press for Success

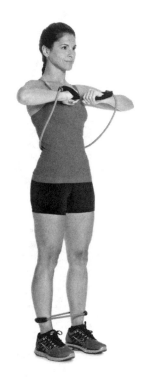

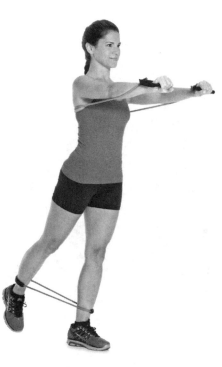

Targets:
Chest, buttocks (pectorals, gluteals)

Do the move:
Stand tall with feet hip-width apart, with a taut resistance band (without handles) around your ankles. Place a second resistance band around your mid-upper back and under your armpits, holding a handle in each hand at chest level, with palms facing down and elbows bent 90 degrees. As you slowly extend your right leg behind you, straighten your arms in front of your chest, wrists in line with forearms. Return to starting position and switch legs. Inhale as you move your leg forward and arms back; exhale as you move arms forward and leg back. Keep toes, knees, hips, and shoulders facing forward, and maintain a straight back and contracted abdominals throughout.

How many?
Start with two sets of 10 repetitions each; work up to three sets of 15.

Challenge yourself:
When you can complete 15 repetitions comfortably, graduate to the next heavier-resistance band.

Two-Timing Curls

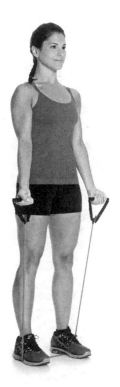 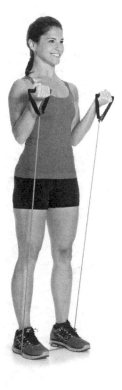

Targets:

Front arms (biceps)

Do the move:

Stand tall with your feet and hands shoulder-width apart. Loop a resistance band under your feet, holding a handle in each hand, palms forward and down at your sides. Curl the bands toward your shoulder, then lower them to starting position. Inhale during the downward movement; exhale as you raise your arms. Keep your toes, knees, hips, and shoulders facing forward, and maintain a straight back and contracted abdominals throughout.

How many?

Start with two sets of 10 repetitions, working up to three sets of 15.

Challenge yourself:

When you can complete 15 repetitions comfortably, graduate to the next heavier-resistance band.

Tummy Tune-Up

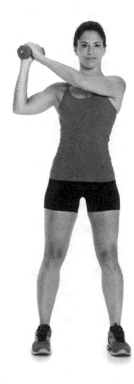 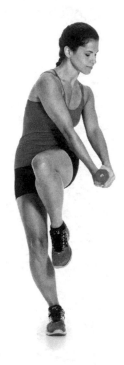

Targets:
Waist, shoulders, hips, buttocks
(obliques, deltoids, hip flexors, gluteals)

Do the move:
Stand tall with your right foot 6 to
12 inches in front of your left. Hold a
5-pound dumbbell over your right shoulder
with both hands. As you slowly pull the
dumbbell diagonally across your body
toward your left hip, twist to your left. At
the same time, lift your left knee toward
your right shoulder. Return to the starting
position and repeat the exercise. Inhale
as you raise your arm; exhale as you lower
it. Finish all your reps on one side before
repeating the exercise on the other side.
Keep toes, knees, hips, and shoulders in
proper alignment, and maintain a straight
back and contracted abdominals.

How many?
Do two sets of 10 repetitions, working
up to three sets of 15.

Challenge yourself:
When you can complete 15 repetitions
comfortably, graduate to the next
heavier weight dumbbell.

Hot to Taut Triceps

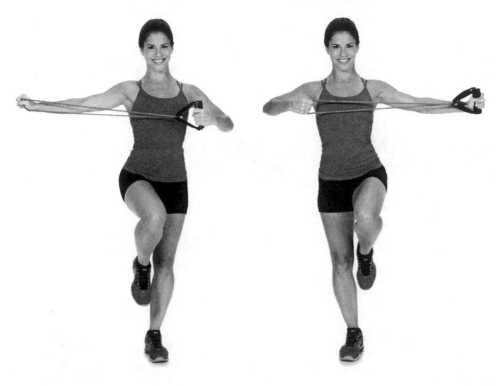

Targets:
Back arms, core, buttocks, hips (triceps, abdominals, gluteals, hip flexors)

Do the move:
Stand tall with your feet hip-width apart and knees soft. Hold a resistance band in a bow-and-arrow position with one arm bent, the other straight, palms at chest level, and wrists in line with forearms. Shift your weight and hop to your right foot while bending your right elbow and extending your left elbow. At the same time, as you balance on your right leg, lift your left knee. Hop onto your left foot and

repeat the exercise. Inhale as you hop; exhale as you bend and extend your arms. Keep your toes, knees, hips, and shoulders facing forward, and maintain a straight back and contracted abdominals.

How many?
Start with two sets of 10 repetitions, working up to three sets of 15.

Challenge yourself:
When you can complete 15 repetitions comfortably, graduate to the next heavier-resistance band.

Rowing Abs

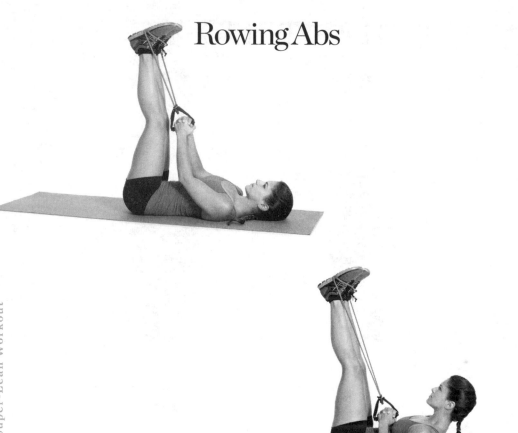

Targets:

Abs, front arms, back, hips (abdominals, biceps, latissimus dorsi, hip flexors)

Do the move:

Wrap a resistance band around your ankles. Lying face-up on the floor, raise both legs, hips bent at 90 degrees with knees above hips. Reach up and grasp handles with both hands, interlacing your fingers. Slowly curl up, lifting your shoulder blades off the floor while pulling the resistance band down by bending your elbows toward your sides. Pause, then slowly return the resistance band to the starting position as you lower your head and shoulders. Inhale during the downward movement; exhale during the upward movement. Maintain a neutral head position, and keep your lower back against the floor.

How many?

Do two sets of 10 repetitions, and work up to three sets of 15.

Challenge yourself:

When you can do 15 repetitions comfortably, graduate to the next heavier-resistance band.

Row, Row, Row Your Back

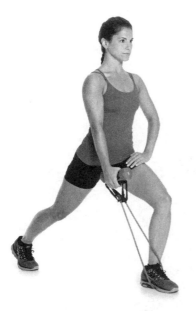

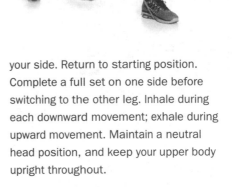

Targets:

Front thighs, back, front arms (quadriceps, latissimus dorsi, biceps)

Do the move:

Stand with feet hip-width apart, with your left foot on the middle of a resistance band, knee bent 90 degrees. Bring your right foot straight back about 2 feet and go up on your toes. Hold a 5-pound dumbbell and both handles in your right hand, and put your left hand on your left thigh to support yourself. Extend your right arm down, palm facing your knee, the resistance band taut. As you slowly lunge your right knee toward the floor, draw the dumbbell and the band up to your side. Return to starting position. Complete a full set on one side before switching to the other leg. Inhale during each downward movement; exhale during upward movement. Maintain a neutral head position, and keep your upper body upright throughout.

How many?

Start with two sets of 10 repetitions and work up to three sets of 15.

Challenge yourself:

When you can complete 15 repetitions comfortably, graduate to the next heavier-resistance band.

Cross-Over Bridge

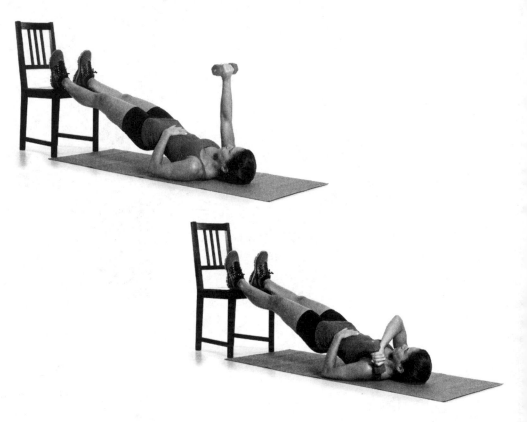

Targets:
Core, rear arms, buttocks, rear thighs
(abdominals, triceps, gluteals, hamstrings)

Do the move:
Lie face-up on the floor and place your
heels on the edge of a chair. With a
3-pound dumbbell in one hand, lift your
hips to form a straight line from your
shoulders to your knees. Extend your right
arm over your right shoulder, and place
your left hand on your abs. Keeping your
upper arm stationary, slowly bend your
right elbow as you lower the dumbbell
toward your left ear, then straighten your

arm. After completing the set, switch to
the other side. Exhale as you raise your
arms; inhale as you lower them. Keep
your shoulder blades on the floor and
your legs straight throughout.

How many?
Do two sets of 10 repetitions, and work
up to three sets of 15.

Challenge yourself:
When you can complete 15 repetitions
comfortably, graduate to the next
heavier dumbbell.

Wind Yourself Up, Calm Yourself Down: Yoga for Every Time of Day

This ancient Indian practice, combining physical poses with deep, even breathing to quiet the mind, can strengthen your muscles and improve your flexibility and balance. Loren Fishman, MD, a specialist in rehabilitation who teaches at Columbia University in New York City and is the author of four books, uses yoga to treat his patients for back pain, arthritis, multiple sclerosis, and even osteoporosis.

We've given you two options: five poses to energize, and five poses to relax. Fcel free to do poses as needed (as an afternoon pick-me-up or a before-bed chill-down), or add them as stretches to your post-strength workouts.

5 Yoga Poses to Energize

Hold each pose through 5 to 10 slow, even breaths, breathing in and out through your nose.

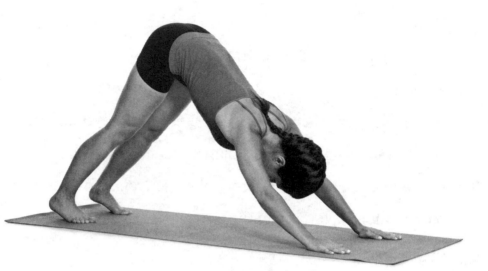

Downward Dog

Often called the all-purpose pose, Downward Dog lengthens the shoulders, spine, and hamstrings. It brings bloodflow to your head and energizes your whole body. Standing with your feet hip-width apart, bend forward until your hands touch the floor and your body makes a V shape. Keeping your arms, back, and legs straight, try to bring your heels toward the floor. Unless you're very flexible, they probably won't touch, but that's not the point anyway. You want to feel the stretch throughout your body.

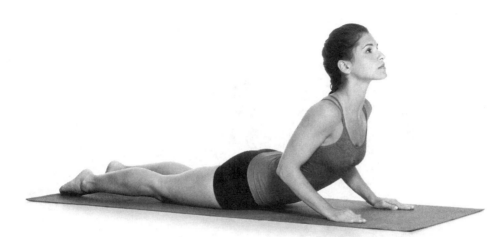

Cobra

Back bends are energizing; this one exercises your arms, opens your chest, and promotes flexibility in your back. Lying face-down on your mat, place your hands, palms down, on either side of your shoulders. Pressing onto your hands, arch your back up, head erect, with your hip bones still touching the floor.

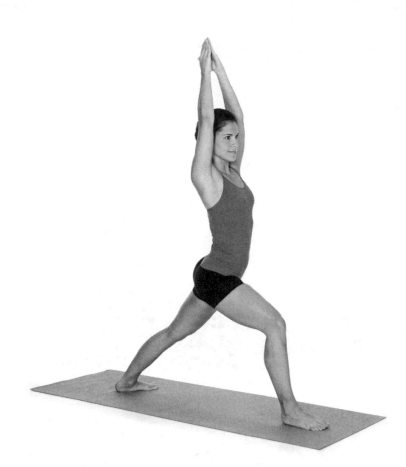

Warrior 1

The Warrior poses call on your strength and balance. Warrior 1 grounds you firmly while at the same time you reach for the sky. Standing in Mountain pose (see page 312), facing forward, place your left foot well behind your right—almost as far as in a runner's squat. With feet flat on the floor, your front foot pointed straight ahead, your back foot at a 45-degree angle, bend your right knee until your thigh is almost horizontal (if you can), keeping your back leg straight. Raise your arms straight overhead, bringing the palms together, and hold your back erect. Reach up as your feet are rooting down into the earth. Bring your left foot forward, returning to Mountain pose, and repeat the exercise on the other side, with your left leg forward and right leg back.

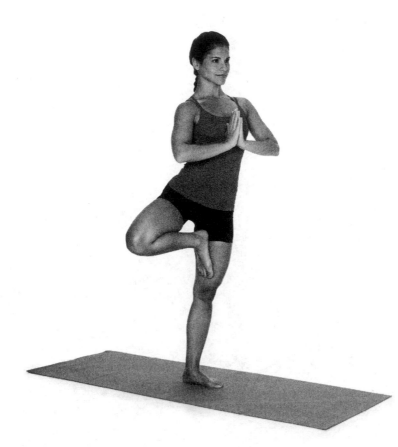

Tree

Balancing poses create energy because we work our core to avoid falling. If you do fall, no worries. Just take a breath and move back into the pose. This is a good beginner's balance. Standing in Mountain pose (see page 312), begin to lift your right foot from the floor, keeping your left leg firm and straight without locking your knee. Rest your right toes on the floor until you feel your balance, then slowly lift them to make a figure 4, resting your foot against the inside of your left leg. It can be above or below your knee but not on the knee. If you feel stable, raise your arms and put your palms together in a prayer pose above your head. Hold for five breaths, if you can, and repeat on the other side.

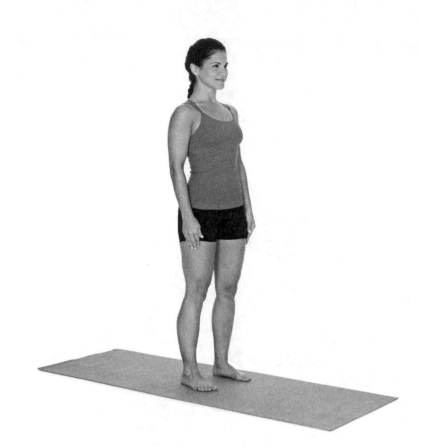

Mountain

The beginning pose in many yoga classes, this is a good place to end our series without losing the energy we've created. Stand with your feet together or hip-width apart (whichever is more comfortable for you), with your arms at your sides. Feel how straight your back is, how evenly distributed your weight is across your feet. Hold your thighs strong, and tuck your tailbone just enough to keep your pelvis neutral. Gaze forward, and breathe slowly and deeply through your nose.

5 Yoga Poses to Relax

Hold each pose through 10 to 20 slow, deep breaths, breathing through your nose.

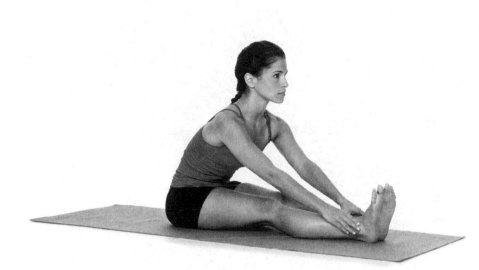

Forward Bend

Just as back bends are energizing, Forward Bends relax you, particularly when done on the floor. Sitting on your mat with your back erect and your legs straight in front of you, slowly lean forward, keeping your back straight and your head up. Let your arms slide down your legs, holding them wherever your fullest stretch is—calf, ankle, or foot. Once you've achieved your stretch, you can allow your upper back and head to relax onto your legs.

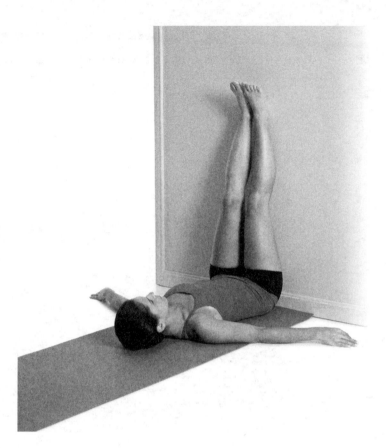

Legs-Up-the-Wall Inversion

Inversions bring blood to your brain and quiet your mind. This effortless inversion will relax you. Lie on your mat with your butt against a wall and your legs up the wall. Place your arms with palms down on either side of your body. Allow your body to soften and melt into the floor.

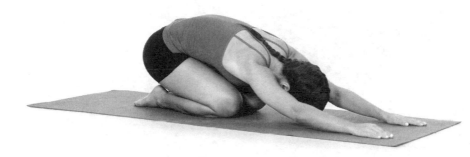

Child's Pose

This asana is often substituted for Downward Dog when a more relaxing pose is wanted. Kneel on your mat with your knees together and your butt resting on your heels. Slowly lower your torso until it is resting on your thighs. If your head doesn't reach the floor, you can place a pillow under it. You can reach forward with your arms, but it's more restful to place them back along your sides, the way a baby sleeps.

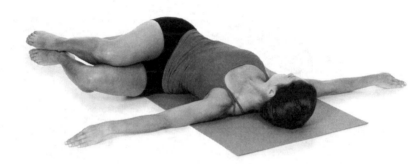

Spinal Twist

Twists can improve digestion by squeezing and stretching your abdominal organs; this one is relatively effortless and relaxing. Lying face-up on your mat with your arms open in a T, palms down, bend your knees into your chest, then lower them to the left, resting your left thigh on the floor if you're flexible enough, but being careful to keep your right shoulder on the floor. Turn your head to the right, and hold as long as comfortable. Raise your legs and reverse the pose, with legs to the right and your head to the left.

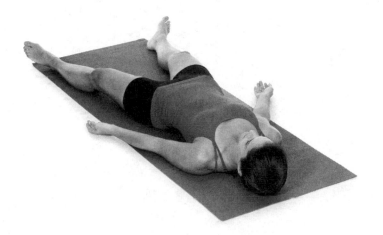

Corpse Pose

Finish your relaxation session with the classic savasana, or meditation, pose. Lie on your mat with your feet about mat's width apart, toes relaxing outward. Place your arms on the floor, palms up, in a comfortable position a small distance from your body. As you lie in Corpse Pose, relax each muscle group in your body—calves, thighs, stomach and buttocks, chest, arms, and neck and head.

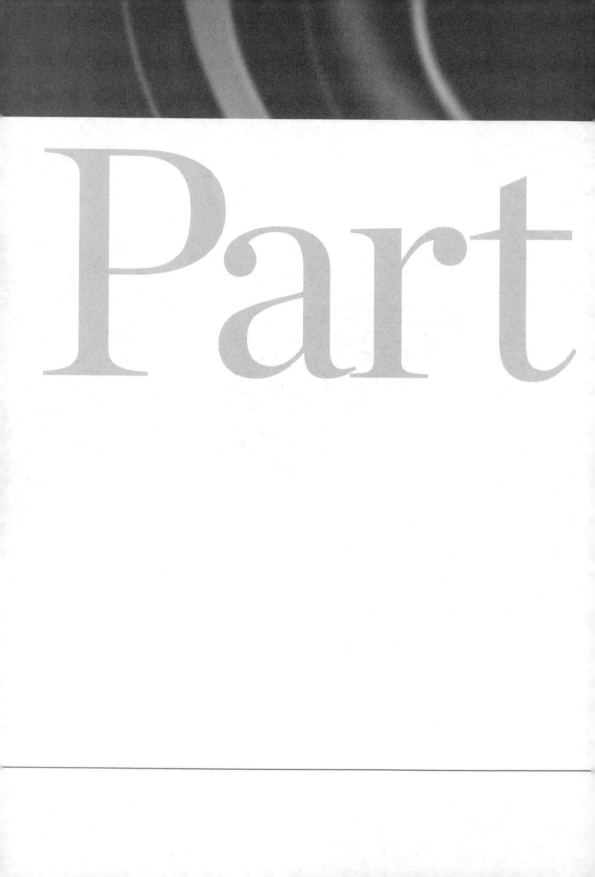

Part

IV

Putting It All Together

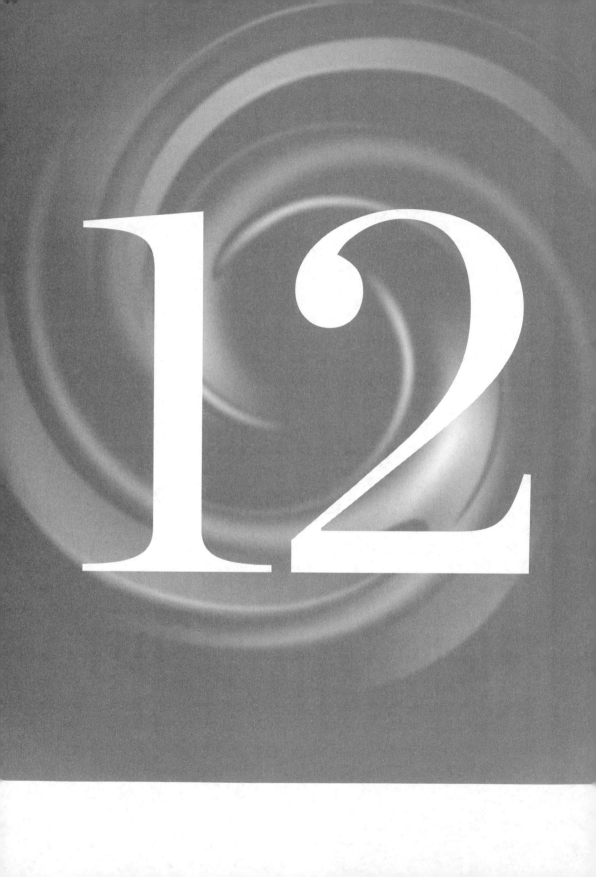

The Ultimate Belly Melt Day

Wake Up! (Same time every day!)

Hit the Reset Button. Within ½ hour and *before* you eat breakfast, do 20 minutes of cardio— walking is fine (5 days a week). Research shows that exercising before breakfast may help you burn fat more efficiently, blunt insulin resistance, and prevent weight gain. In the study, a pre-breakfast workout negated the usual damage done by unhealthy high-fat meals. And if you can get outside, even better. By exposing your body to light early in the morning, it naturally resets itself to a healthier sleep/wake cycle.

Time to Eat. The alarm clock has stirred more than you—it woke up the hormone ghrelin, the "feed me" hormone that's made in your stomach. Ignore ghrelin and not only will you set the stage for cravings later on (he just keeps getting angrier if you don't feed him), but skipping breakfast sends your natural cycle into a hormonal tailspin. Ghrelin has also nudged awake neuropeptide Y (NPY), a gut hormone that regulates appetite and the desire for carbohydrates. A small serving of healthy carbs—such as the vegetables in your omelet or whole wheat toast—will keep NPY from nagging you all morning and triggering those 10:00 doughnut cravings. So within an hour of waking up, treat yourself to a relatively big breakfast that mixes complex carbs (like whole grain bread or cereal) and protein (eggs, egg whites, fat-free milk, low-fat cheese). The whole grains and protein slow your blood sugar's rise and suppress ghrelin longer. Why have a big breakfast? Because the food you eat in the morning has a higher satiety level—meaning it makes you feel fuller—than the food you eat at night.

After you eat (at any time), levels of leptin, an appetite-suppressing hormone made by your fat cells, go up, and that tells NPY to simmer down. And as food is digested in your gut, your body produces a chemical, cholecystokinin (CCK), that acts synergistically with leptin to turn off your appetite and tell you you're full.

Hit the Reset Button. Before breakfast—and every meal—drink two 8-ounce glasses of water. A study at Virginia Tech published in the journal *Obesity* found that people who drank this amount before breakfast, lunch, and dinner lost 5 pounds more (and kept it off) than those who didn't.

Midmorning

Time to Eat. Ghrelin begins to rise a couple of hours before lunch to remind you to eat (as if you needed a reminder). In animal studies, mice and rats start exhibiting "food anticipatory behavior," such as running in their wheels and checking the food dispenser, when the ghrelin starts pumping. Humans usually find themselves wandering to the vending machines. (See, we told you those cravings weren't your fault!) Ghrelin turns off when you eat—particularly carbs and protein—so it's okay to have a small combo snack now. Carbs shut off ghrelin pretty quickly, and protein keeps it turned off longer. Since everyone has a different schedule, time this snack at the midpoint between your breakfast and lunch. (So if you ate breakfast at 8:00, and you plan to lunch at noon, snack at 10:00.)

Hit the Reset Button. Don't let 4 hours go by without eating. Eating even "a little something" stimulates the secretion of a hormone called peptide YY-36, which reduces ghrelin production and shuts off your appetite. Never eat a carb without a protein. Protein slows digestion and helps keep blood sugar stable, so you'll feel full and satisfied, and fatigue won't make you succumb to bad-for-you goodies.

Lunch

Time to Eat. Ghrelin is up again, but so is a new hunger hormone—galanin. Galanin makes you want to eat fat; it starts up at lunchtime and peaks in the evening. However, eating a high-fat lunch isn't a good idea. Fatty foods don't suppress the "eat more" effects of ghrelin as well as carbs and proteins do (actually, hardly at all). Plus, dietary fat causes you to produce more galanin, which then tells you to eat more fat, and a vicious cycle starts.

This is no time to have that big bowl of pasta, either. Carbs produce a huge blood sugar spike that's followed by a precipitous drop, which can leave you tired and hungry by midafternoon. They also raise levels of the amino acid tryptophan. The body uses it to make melatonin, the sleep hormone. Ghrelin will shut off when you eat, and leptin goes up. But you'll feel fullest and most alert if you have a lunch of carbs and protein together.

The key to lunch isn't just the foods, but eating at the same time each day. As you can see from this complex dance of hormones, working through the lunch hour, only to wolf down something at 3:00, sends them into a tizzy, which subsequently whacks out your circadian cycle, as well as your body's natural hunger cycle. (Don't forget your two glasses of water beforehand!)

Midafternoon

Hit the Reset Button. Take a nap. Thirty minutes or less has been shown to energize your body without ruining your sleep cycle for the night.

Time to Eat. Nap not possible? Have a turkey roll-up instead. The amino acid tyrosine, found in protein, promotes alertness, making that your best midafternoon pick-me-up. (By the way, that slump is not in your head. It's at this point that your body temperature drops, as does blood sugar, triggered by insulin secretion after your lunch. Leptin also hits bottom. That's why you can't stop thinking about Ho Hos.) Protein also raises levels of the brain chemical dopamine, which is in charge of pleasure, as well as norepinephrine, an adrenal hormone secreted to give you sudden energy when you're under stress. It's a little like your body's own shot of espresso, making you feel perky again. Speaking of coffee, if you really need a quick blast of alertness, now's the last time to do it. Coffee after 4:00 p.m. has been shown to foil circadian rhythms and may keep you from falling asleep tonight.

Early Evening

Hit the Reset Button. Now is the time to do your strength-training and stretching workouts, as well as any more intense cardio. In one study, subjects built 22 percent more muscle by working out in the late afternoon/early evening than morning exercisers. This is when your body temperature is at its highest, so your body performs at its peak, which also protects it against injury. Exercising at the same time every day also helps stabilize your circadian rhythms, so that set of lunges you're doing now will help you sleep better tonight—and feel more awake tomorrow.

Dinner

Time to Eat. Your body is producing ghrelin and galanin again. Ghrelin is telling you to eat, and galanin is urging you to eat fat because it wants to make sure you have enough calories on board so you don't wake up at night. This is a great time to load up on healthy fats like olive oil and fish oil (which, as you've seen, is one of our Sleep and Sleek Foods, because it promotes sleep and resets your body's rhythm on its own). While we want you to eat enough to stay asleep, don't overdo it: Studies show increased weight loss when more calories are consumed in the a.m. than in the p.m. And eating at night throws off circadian rhythms.

Late Evening/Bedtime

Time to Eat. Nighttime carbs create tryptophan, which promotes good sleep patterns. (One study found that even high-glycemic carbs—sweet things that raise your blood sugar—can help you fall asleep faster.) That surge in tryptophan helps your brain produce serotonin, the feel-good chemical that also triggers your body to make melatonin, the sleep hormone. Overnight, your body will tap into your fat stores for fuel so you don't wake up jonesing for a midnight snack. And you have a fail-safe system on board: The appetite suppressant leptin is at its peak after midnight.

Hit the Reset Button. Step away from the iPad, the BlackBerry, the iPhone, and the laptop. . . . Studies have found that the bluish light they emit actually is even more disruptive to sleep than full-spectrum light. In fact, about ½ hour before bedtime, turn down all the lights and do something calming—meditate, read, take a bath, sip sleep-promoting chamomile or passionflower tea—in dim light. Your body can produce the sleep hormone melatonin only under cover of darkness, so this period before darkness will have you ready to nod off once you hit the sheets.

Go to Sleep! Same time every night!

Tackling the Cycle Busters

You know this drill from your past: Whenever you try to slim down, sooner or later something comes along, and whammo, the wheels come off the tracks. This is when the negative self-talk kicks in—without regard to what might have been behind the derailing. You tell yourself that you just don't have the willpower to stick to any-thing, that it's your fault, or that you don't have what it takes to be thin and healthy. As in, here you go—again.

But that kind of thinking couldn't be more misguided—what's more, it deprives you of the opportunity to examine the other influences that may be interfering with your resolve. Willpower gets the blame, but the truth is, there are stealth internal and external forces that are really at work. And as you've probably figured out by now, they have to do with your cycle.

Anything that affects your body clock can subtly affect your ability to lose weight. Time changes, seasonal changes, chronic pain, schedule changes. Here's a rundown of the cycle busters and what you can do to minimize the damage.

Seasonal Change

Back in Chapter 1, we looked at the different rhythms that govern us—circadian, ultradian, infradian, diurnal, and nocturnal. We left one off the list: circannual, the rhythms that reflect the changing length of days throughout the year. After June's summer solstice, days start shortening. And the farther north of the equator you are, the shorter your days become.

Then, when daylight saving time ends in November, the shorter, darker days that ensue can trigger depression—a condition known as seasonal affective disorder (the appropriately dubbed SAD). And that's bad news for your mood—not to mention your waistline. According to scientists at Finland's National Institute for Health and Welfare, with seasonal light changes come sleep disturbances that can trigger negative thoughts and low self-esteem—both of which are known diet saboteurs. And there's more: The changes bump up your appetite, making it harder to stick to your commitment to eat more healthfully. So it's not just in your head that you want to munch more when the days get shorter.

An estimated 50 percent of Americans who live in the northern half of the country (which starts roughly at the northern border of Virginia in the east and slices through the country to San Francisco in the west) are sensitive to seasonal light changes. If you're among them, less light in the fall and winter translates to a vicious cycle diet-wise—you become less active and tend to crave carbs at night.

Think hibernation and you begin to get the drift of what your body is trying to do. To our ancestors, shutting down and chubbing up for the winter meant the difference between life and death—winter really was the killing season for humans. Cooler, shorter fall days signaled that it was time for people to bulk up, store whatever food they could find (starchy roots and summer-fatted animals), and hunker down close to the hearth to await spring.

We're so hardwired to this seasonal pull to slow down that our bodies try to re-create a semi-hibernation as winter ensues. Only now, "hibernating" runs counter to our fast-paced lives—we have jobs and multilevel responsibilities that leave no time for cozy hearth napping, to say nothing of mega-carb and fat loading. What once was a human survival strategy has become the syndrome called SAD.

The symptoms of SAD can range from cases of the blues that are so subtle that you may not even be aware you're affected, to severe depression that affects your ability to function.

Light Up Your Life

Though you can't argue with a circadian clock that was set 50,000 or so years ago, you can reset it. All it takes is timed doses of bright light during the day. And here's the good news: This isn't one of those therapies you sit through for weeks before it works; just 20 minutes of light sitting can give your winter blues the heave-ho.

Results of a 2009 study by some of the leading light-therapy researchers in the country showed that just 20 minutes of exposure to bright-light therapy improved people's depression scores immediately. And they felt even better after 40 minutes of exposure. In a 2010 University of Rochester study, when researchers treated 51 people with SAD with bright-light therapy,

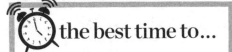

the best time to...

GET A SKIN CANCER CHECK

Winter is the best time for your annual top-to-toes checkup for a simple reason: Your skin is probably lighter in this season, making it easier to spot moles or other lesions that may warrant a biopsy.

nearly half of them were symptom free after 7 days of treatment.

That's important to know, because depression and weight gain are inexorably linked. A 2010 study conducted at Brigham Young University in Utah showed that middle-aged women had a 59 percent greater risk of gaining weight if they were depressed than women who weren't depressed. In a 2011 Japanese study, when researchers followed a group of 1,730 workers for 4 years, they found that depressed workers gained almost 9 pounds more during the study than happier workers.

Truth is, "being depressed actually makes you gain weight," said Belinda L. Needham, PhD, assistant professor of sociology at the University of Alabama in Birmingham, in a much-reported 2010 study. She noted that young people who are depressed tend to exercise less and eat more. Even depression treatments can bust your diet: Perversely, antidepressants have a tendency to make people gain weight, Dr. Needham said. In her study, she and a team of researchers examined data from 5,115 people, ages 18 to 30. Participants agreed to have their depression symptoms, BMI, and waist circumference checked over the course of 15 years.

You'd think that gaining weight (which nearly everyone in Dr. Needham's study managed to do over the 15-year study) is a for-sure depression trigger, but you'd be wrong. Turns out, the folks who were heavier at the start of the study didn't become more depressed by its end. Nor did they pack on as much belly fat as did the people who were depressed. Instead, those with higher depression scores plumped up—in the study's 20-year checkup, people who were depressed had bigger waist measurements than people who weren't depressed.

Light therapy may also help you with the other problem that happens when the days get shorter and darker: a drop-off in exercise. If your mental outlook is healthier, you're more likely to stick with your exercise regimen, which will probably have to come indoors a bit more during this time of year.

So let's recap: Too little light can lead to depression. Depression can lead to weight gain. Light therapy treats depression and can kick-start you back into your BMD groove again. See "Come to the Light" on page 64 for how to use light therapy.

Pain's a Sleep Killer

If you're in pain, getting a good night's sleep may be the impossible dream. And you're not alone—the number of people who say that pain interrupts their sleep is on the rise. Sixty-six percent of people who have chronic pain—one in five younger adults and one in two older adults—have trouble sleeping.

Certain pain problems have a special ability to wreck your refreshing sleep. Think back pain, headaches, and facial pain (caused by temporomandibular joint, or TMJ, syndrome). Then there's the allover aching of fibromyalgia and the joint pain—knees and hips are particular targets—that arthritis causes. In women, menstrual cramps and abdominal pain make the pain-that-wakes-you-up list, too.

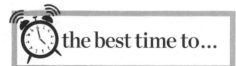 the best time to...

HAVE YOUR CHOLESTEROL TESTED

Run the test twice a year, during the summer, and again in December, when cholesterol peaks. If you average the two readings, you'll have the best picture of your cholesterol level year-round.

The pain/poor sleep connection might seem obvious, but it's more nuanced than you might expect. See, when you first experience pain at night, you'll likely be able to sleep right through it. But when pain becomes entrenched, sleep becomes elusive, and a vicious cycle begins. Being blasted awake and in pain one night makes you fear a replay the next night, so you sleep less soundly in anticipation. That makes it easy for even less intense pain to shake you out of slumber. Pretty soon, your chronic pain has turned you into a chronic insomniac.

What's the solution? If your pain is relatively minor, you may be able to sleep through it if you follow the sleep hygiene suggestions on page 47 faithfully. But if those tips don't help, you'll need to discuss your situation with a health care professional. It could be that your pain is being under-treated: You might be reluctant to ask your doctor to treat pain aggressively because women are often shy about asking for the strong pain medications they need—and some doctors just plain don't take pain seriously enough.

Nondrug options for pain treatment include physical therapy, cognitive behavior therapy, guided imagery, biofeedback, hypnotherapy, and

HOW TO SLEEP ON A BAD BACK

If your back cries out during the night, it could be the way that you're sleeping. These easy fixes will make you and your spine more comfortable.

Belly sleepers. If you sleep face-down, you're straining your back. Position a pillow under your hips and lower belly and another under your head—but lose that one if you feel any lower back strain.

Back sleepers. Tuck a pillow under your knees to help maintain the natural curve of your lower spine. Roll up a towel tightly and put it under the small of your back for extra support, and use a pillow under your neck.

Side sleepers. Pull your legs up toward your chest and wedge a pillow between your legs. A full-length body pillow works really well for this position—which also helps ease hip pain.

progressive muscle relaxation. But these natural approaches don't work for everyone—and they take precious time to work. Bottom line: Don't stiff-upper-lip pain that wrecks your sleep. Talk to your doctor about it, and remember that asking for help isn't a sign of weakness.

Shift Work

When other people's night is your day (and vice versa), the clash between daily life and your body's natural cycles is even more intense. If you work a night shift or, for that matter, any shift that deviates from the typical 9-to-5 life, sleeping well may not come easily to you. It's not hard to understand why 30 percent of shift workers say that they feel exhausted on the job and yet have trouble sleeping during the day. Shift work disorder is linked to poor performance (which may cause on-the-job safety lapses), accidents outside of work, heart disease, diabetes, ulcers, stomach problems, depression, and even fertility issues.

And that's not all. There's a clear link between obesity and shift work. Reasons include poor diet and not enough activity, for starters, but it's likely that other factors are involved. For one thing, shift work seems to lower leptin levels—the hormone that makes you feel full. So it's possible that shift workers feel hungrier, and as a result eat more, than day workers. Healthful food options are likely to be more of a problem, especially at "lunch" time, and vending machines may be a shift worker's only available food source. Since depression is linked to shift work, that may play a part in weight problems, too.

Studies at Harvard have found that people who sleep during the day and are up at night—and eat accordingly—quickly develop serious biochemical changes that may predispose them to sleep, metabolic, and cardiovascular problems, including insomnia, diabetes, and heart disease. For example, in one study of 10 adults who ate and slept at all phases of the circadian cycle in a lab, the volunteers slept poorly. Their cortisol cycle—which usually rises in the morning to help wake us—was reversed. They also had higher blood pressure, blood glucose, and insulin, and lower secretions of the appetite suppressant leptin. Three of the study participants actually developed symptoms of prediabetes during the study. And they were only "working" the third shift for 10 days.

Here's why: When you're a shift worker, your natural circadian rhythms aren't in sync with your unnatural work patterns. As far as sleep is concerned, most shift workers experience problems with insomnia—it may take you anywhere from 1 to 4 hours to nod off when it's time for bed. And if your shift is at night or in the early morning, you're likely to have the most trouble sleeping.

We do have some good news: The Belly Melt Diet program is perfectly suited for shift workers. While we do require you to eat, sleep, and exercise on a regular cycle, the great part is that *you* get to set that cycle. It's not based on a clock's time of day—it's based on your time of day.

And if you don't believe us, then we beg you to read Erin Posten's story on page 336. Erin works a second shift, crafted the Belly Melt Diet program to her schedule, and lost 18 pounds in just 5 weeks. She also said that her energy doubled, and she slept better than ever, too.

Working odd hours can be difficult, but losing weight doesn't have to be. Here's how to do it, on your time.

Stick to a schedule. The BMD schedule (see Chapter 5) can work for you. If you get up at 11:00 a.m., that's the time when you walk, and then eat your breakfast. You have your snack 2 hours later, and then lunch, and so on. You can even plan your workout for after work, just as you would if you worked a day shift. And whatever you do, go to bed when you need to. You still need 8 hours of sleep each day. You can use the tips in Chapter 3 to help you get a good night's sleep; they work for day or night. If you stick to a strict schedule (and, say, don't try to live the life of a 9-to-5er on weekends), your body rhythms will adjust and that will become your normal.

Ask for help at home. When your night is your family's day, it can be hard to get the sleep you need. You need quiet, uninterrupted sack time. Let your family know how important it is for you to get proper rest, and work out a schedule that fits your needs as well as theirs.

Take a power nap. Studies have shown that taking a nap for just 20 minutes on your lunch break will improve your reaction time and alertness.

Use bright light. If at all possible, expose yourself to bright light as much as possible during your shift. Consider buying a portable light unit, and do your work close to it—or use it while on your lunch break. (See "Come to the Light" on page 64 for information on light systems.)

Don shades. Wearing dark or amber sunglasses to shield your eyes from bright light toward the end of your night shift and while you're traveling home will help keep your rhythms in line. (See page 46 for information on special glasses.)

Make coffee your shift buddy. The American Academy of Sleep Medicine recommends using caffeine to keep your alertness at peak levels during your shift—and at least one study confirms its value. When workers drank coffee before and during the first part of their night shift, they were much less sleepy and rated themselves as 25 percent more alert. What's more, a

Fasting Travel

We don't recommend fasting on the Belly Melt Diet, unless you're a long-distance traveler trying to avoid jet lag. If you're crossing several time zones, a 2009 study by researchers at Harvard Medical School and Beth Israel Deaconess Medical Center in Boston suggests that fasting for 16 hours will reset your food clock, and that will override your light-sensitive SCN, the master clock that controls your body timing (and which is what triggers jet lag). In other words, you'll adjust quickly to the new time zone by not eating until you get to your destination and then eating on that schedule. Voilà—no jet lag!

(continued on page 338)

My Belly Melt

"One of the guys I walk with at work now tells me I'm too fast!"

Erin Posten

AGE: 33

POUNDS LOST: 18.4 in 35 days

POUNDS LOST IN 3-DAY RESET: 4.5

ALLOVER INCHES LOST: 8.25

INCHES FROM WAIST LOST: 4.75

BODY FAT LOST: 1.6 percent

Erin Posten can hardly believe the scale—she's lost more than 18 pounds in just 5 weeks. But she knows it's true when she looks in a mirror or fingers her suddenly way-too-roomy waistband. Victory is especially sweet because Erin faced an extra obstacle in her path to weight loss: her job. Working the second shift, from 4:00 p.m. to midnight, made it harder to establish a good, healthy rhythm. She had to create a routine that suited her life. BMD gave her that routine.

After

Success Story

Sleep is the secret weapon in making her schedule work. "Once I started going to bed earlier—at 3:00 a.m.—everything started to flow," Erin says. She had been getting only 5 or 6 hours of sleep; now that she's sleeping a solid 8 hours every night, her energy is up and her appetite is down.

Her mealtimes may be odd, but the BMD eating plan keeps her satisfied and cures her cravings. Erin was so satisfied by the 1,200-calorie diet in the Reset phase that the Phase 2 food seemed like too much to eat. "I was never hungry," she recalls. At first, drinking so much water felt weird, but soon she grew to depend on it: "I felt like I couldn't eat without my water; it really made me feel fuller."

Instead of walking in the morning (when she is sound asleep), Erin does two 20-minute walks on a path at her workplace during breaks. "I walk with two co-workers, and we almost never miss a day." She does her strength training after work, at 1:30 a.m., just like normal shifters.

At 5 weeks on the plan, Erin's energy has doubled. Want proof? "One of the guys I walk with at work now tells me I'm too fast," she says, laughing. Before the program, she dragged after dinner. Now she's got energy to spare. "There was one time in Phase 2 when my energy lagged. I increased my exercise and got my energy back.

"I love the routine, knowing what I'm supposed to do," she continues. "It's manageable." Because Erin and her mom, Karen (profile on page 112), are on the plan together, they encourage each other. And the results are great: "People say I behave a lot more positively. I'm more awake, and I'm slimming down."

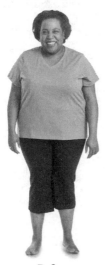

Before

recent review of studies shows that compared with a placebo, coffee improved shift workers' performance, memory, and attention. But . . .

. . . Don't drink it too late. To avoid ruining your sleep, never drink caffeine within 5 hours of your bedtime. Studies also find that most shift workers do just the opposite—drink caffeine late in their shift, which thwarts their efforts to sleep later!

Try melatonin. In studies, people who took 1.8 to 6 milligrams of melatonin just before going to bed (during the day, if you work the night shift) slept longer.

Appendix

The Belly Melt Diet
Journal

Through reading this book, you have discovered an unbeatable program to banish belly fat, eliminate sleepless nights, and halt out-of-control cravings. Now it's time to personalize the plan to work specifically for you. Keeping a journal can help you map out the cycles to which your body is currently synced, and in no time at all, you'll have made huge steps in resetting your many internal clocks. In the following pages, you will find 3 days' worth of journal pages for the Reset phase (with a weigh-in sheet so you can see your quick-start results!) and a week's worth of pages that you can photocopy for the Reshape phase. Photocopying these pages will allow you to keep your own journal for 5 weeks (the duration for which our test panelists pioneered the program) or longer as you adjust to the Belly Melt Diet program and get the results you want.

Here's how the journal pages are set up: On page 341, you will find a Starting Stats page where you can record your starting weight and circumference measurements before beginning the program. Next come the daily logs. The first few questions are designed to help you track your meals, including what foods you consume and what time you have each meal, with the option to catalog how many servings or calories you've had. We have included basic guidelines for each phase of the plan in Chapters 7

(Reset) and 8 (Reshape), and you can find serving size guidelines on page 118. Logging this information over a few weeks will help you see the cause-and-effect relationship between changing your diet and the sliding numbers on the scale.

In addition to a food log, we also provide space to track your sleep and exercise habits, as well as to rate your craving and mood levels. The last section, Cycle Watch, is where you can track the time of year and where you are in your menstrual cycle, if applicable. This will help you become mindful of patterns and problems as you work toward getting back in sync with your body's own rhythms.

At the end of each set of Reset and Reshape journal pages, you will see a measurements page. On this page, you can weigh in, record how many inches you've lost that week, and take a moment to assess how another week of the program has affected your overall health and well-being.

After a few days of practice, you'll find that keeping a journal is a cinch! Before you know it, eating right, staying active, and getting the sleep you deserve will naturally become your new lifestyle.

Starting Stats

Before you start the program, take your starting measurements so that you'll be able to see changes in your body in real time! As the weeks go by, you can compare the falling numbers on your most recent weekly check-in page to the chart below. Seeing the numbers go in the right direction can help keep you motivated—and if the numbers aren't moving as much as you'd like, this info can cue you to modify the program to maximize your results.

	Today	In 12 Weeks
HEIGHT		
WEIGHT		
BODY MASS INDEX (BMI)		
CHEST		
WAIST		
HIPS (AT FULLEST PART)		
LEFT THIGH		
RIGHT THIGH		
LEFT BICEPS		
RIGHT BICEPS		

How to calculate your BMI: Multiply your weight in pounds by 703. Divide that number by your height in inches. Divide that number by your height in inches again. Or to make things easier, plug in your numbers at Prevention.com/bmi to use our online BMI calculator.

Circumference measurements: To get the most accurate measurements, we recommend having a spouse or friend help. Be sure to stand up straight, with your shoulders back and arms relaxed, and measure your limbs and torso using these starting points:

- Chest: the fullest point of your bust
- Waist: the narrowest part of your torso (usually about 2 inches above your belly button)
- Hips: the fullest part, with the tape measure evenly parallel to the ground all the way around your hips
- Arms and thighs: the fullest part of each, when relaxed, with arms hanging down and feet shoulder-width apart

Reset

DATE: HOURS SLEPT:

Rate quality of sleep: (*1 being poorest and 10 being best*)

1   2   3   4   5   6   7   8   9   10

Breakfast | TIME | _____

_____

_____

_____

Total Calories or Servings _____

Midmorning Snack | TIME | _____

_____

_____

Total Calories or Servings _____

Lunch | TIME | _____

_____

_____

_____

Total Calories or Servings _____

Midafternoon Snack | TIME | _____

_____

_____

Total Calories or Servings _____

Dinner | TIME | _____

_____

_____

_____

Total Calories or Servings _____

Nighttime Snack `TIME` _____

_____

Total Calories or Servings _____

WORKOUT

Cardio/Walk `TIME` `DURATION` _____

_____

Strength workout `TIME` _____

_____

Rate strength of cravings throughout day
(1 being very strong and 10 being no cravings at all):

1   2   3   4   5   6   7   8   9   10

Rate overall mood _(1 being poorest and 10 being best):_

1   2   3   4   5   6   7   8   9   10

Additional comments/notes/questions: _____

_____

_____

⊚ Cycle Watch

Day of cycle _(Comments):_ _____

_____

Season _(Comments):_ _____

_____

Reset

DATE: _____ HOURS SLEPT: _____

Rate quality of sleep: (*1 being poorest and 10 being best*)

1   2   3   4   5   6   7   8   9   10

Breakfast | TIME | _____
_____
_____
_____

Total Calories or Servings _____

Midmorning Snack | TIME | _____
_____
_____

Total Calories or Servings _____

Lunch | TIME | _____
_____
_____
_____

Total Calories or Servings _____

Midafternoon Snack | TIME | _____
_____
_____

Total Calories or Servings _____

Dinner | TIME | _____
_____
_____
_____

Total Calories or Servings _____

Nighttime Snack | TIME | _____

_____

Total Calories or Servings _____

WORKOUT

Cardio/Walk | TIME | | DURATION | _____

Strength workout | TIME | _____

Rate strength of cravings throughout day
(1 being very strong and 10 being no cravings at all):

1   2   3   4   5   6   7   8   9   10

Rate overall mood *(1 being poorest and 10 being best):*

1   2   3   4   5   6   7   8   9   10

Additional comments/notes/questions: _____

_____

_____

Cycle Watch

Day of cycle *(Comments):* _____

_____

Season *(Comments):* _____

_____

Reset

DATE: _____ HOURS SLEPT: _____

Rate quality of sleep: *(1 being poorest and 10 being best)*

1   2   3   4   5   6   7   8   9   10

Breakfast | TIME | _____

_____

_____

_____

Total Calories or Servings _____

Midmorning Snack | TIME | _____

_____

Total Calories or Servings _____

Lunch | TIME | _____

_____

_____

_____

Total Calories or Servings _____

Midafternoon Snack | TIME | _____

_____

Total Calories or Servings _____

Dinner | TIME | _____

_____

_____

_____

Total Calories or Servings _____

Nighttime Snack TIME

_____

Total Calories or Servings _____

WORKOUT
Cardio/Walk TIME DURATION _____

Strength workout TIME _____

Rate strength of cravings throughout day
(1 being very strong and 10 being no cravings at all):

1   2   3   4   5   6   7   8   9   10

Rate overall mood _(1 being poorest and 10 being best):_

1   2   3   4   5   6   7   8   9   10

Additional comments/notes/questions: _____

_____

_____

◎ Cycle Watch

Day of cycle _(Comments):_ _____

_____

Season _(Comments):_ _____

_____

Reset Check-In

WEIGHT	
CHEST	
WAIST	
HIPS (AT FULLEST PART)	
LEFT THIGH	
RIGHT THIGH	
LEFT BICEPS	
RIGHT BICEPS	

Overall Weekly Energy Level
(1 = I wish I was still in bed, 10 = I'm like a kid in a candy store)

1   2   3   4   5   6   7   8   9   10

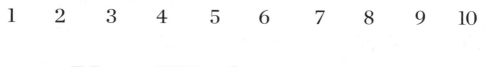

Your Week in Review

Use this space to record any additional thoughts or feelings or to look back on the last couple of days and mark your success on the Belly Melt Diet.

_____

_____

_____

_____

_____

_____

_____

_____

_____

_____

_____

Week ___ Reshape Day 1

Rate quality of sleep: (*1 being poorest and 10 being best*)

1   2   3   4   5   6   7   8   9   10

Breakfast | TIME | _____

_____

_____

_____

Total Calories or Servings _____

Midmorning Snack | TIME | _____

_____

Total Calories or Servings _____

Lunch | TIME | _____

_____

_____

_____

Total Calories or Servings _____

Midafternoon Snack | TIME | _____

_____

Total Calories or Servings _____

Dinner | TIME | _____

_____

_____

_____

Total Calories or Servings _____

Nighttime Snack | TIME |

Total Calories or Servings _____

WORKOUT

Cardio/Walk | TIME | | DURATION |

Strength workout | TIME |

Rate strength of cravings throughout day
(1 being very strong and 10 being no cravings at all):

1   2   3   4   5   6   7   8   9   10

Rate overall mood *(1 being poorest and 10 being best):*

1   2   3   4   5   6   7   8   9   10

Additional comments/notes/questions: _____

Cycle Watch

Day of cycle *(Comments):* _____

Season *(Comments):* _____

DATE: HOURS SLEPT:

Rate quality of sleep: (1 being poorest and 10 being best)

1   2   3   4   5   6   7   8   9   10

Breakfast | TIME |

_____

_____

_____

Total Calories or Servings _____

Midmorning Snack | TIME |

_____

Total Calories or Servings _____

Lunch | TIME |

_____

_____

Total Calories or Servings _____

Midafternoon Snack | TIME |

_____

Total Calories or Servings _____

Dinner | TIME |

_____

_____

_____

Total Calories or Servings _____

Nighttime Snack | TIME | _____ |

_____

Total Calories or Servings _____

WORKOUT

Cardio/Walk | TIME | | DURATION | _____

_____

Strength workout | TIME | _____

_____

Rate strength of cravings throughout day
(1 being very strong and 10 being no cravings at all):

| 1 | 2 | 3 | 4 | 5 | 6 | 7 | 8 | 9 | 10 |

Rate overall mood *(1 being poorest and 10 being best):*

| 1 | 2 | 3 | 4 | 5 | 6 | 7 | 8 | 9 | 10 |

Additional comments/notes/questions: _____

_____

Cycle Watch

Day of cycle *(Comments):* _____

_____

Season *(Comments):* _____

_____

Week __ Reshape Day 3

DATE: HOURS SLEPT:

Rate quality of sleep: (*1 being poorest and 10 being best*)

1   2   3   4   5   6   7   8   9   10

Breakfast | TIME | _____

_____

_____

Total Calories or Servings _____

Midmorning Snack | TIME | _____

_____

Total Calories or Servings _____

Lunch | TIME | _____

_____

_____

Total Calories or Servings _____

Midafternoon Snack | TIME | _____

_____

Total Calories or Servings _____

Dinner | TIME | _____

_____

_____

_____

Total Calories or Servings _____

Nighttime Snack | TIME | | _____

_____

_____

Total Calories or Servings _____

WORKOUT

Cardio/Walk | TIME | | DURATION | | _____

_____

Strength workout | TIME | | _____

_____

Rate strength of cravings throughout day
(1 being very strong and 10 being no cravings at all):

1   2   3   4   5   6   7   8   9   10

Rate overall mood *(1 being poorest and 10 being best):*

1   2   3   4   5   6   7   8   9   10

Additional comments/notes/questions: _____

_____

_____

◎ Cycle Watch _____

Day of cycle *(Comments):* _____

_____

Season *(Comments):* _____

_____

Week ___ Reshape Day 4

Rate quality of sleep: (*1 being poorest and 10 being best*)

1   2   3   4   5   6   7   8   9   10

Breakfast | TIME | _____

_____

_____

_____

Total Calories or Servings _____

Midmorning Snack | TIME | _____

_____

Total Calories or Servings _____

Lunch | TIME | _____

_____

_____

_____

Total Calories or Servings _____

Midafternoon Snack | TIME | _____

_____

Total Calories or Servings _____

Dinner | TIME | _____

_____

_____

_____

_____

Total Calories or Servings _____

Nighttime Snack `TIME` _____ _____

_____

_____

Total Calories or Servings _____

WORKOUT

Cardio/Walk `TIME` | `DURATION` _____

_____

Strength workout `TIME` _____

_____

Rate strength of cravings throughout day
(1 being very strong and 10 being no cravings at all):

1   2   3   4   5   6   7   8   9   10

Rate overall mood *(1 being poorest and 10 being best):*

1   2   3   4   5   6   7   8   9   10

Additional comments/notes/questions: _____

_____

_____

Cycle Watch

Day of cycle *(Comments):* _____

_____

Season *(Comments):* _____

_____

Week ___ Reshape Day 5

Rate quality of sleep: (*1 being poorest and 10 being best*)

1   2   3   4   5   6   7   8   9   10

Breakfast | TIME |

Total Calories or Servings _____

Midmorning Snack | TIME |

Total Calories or Servings _____

Lunch | TIME |

Total Calories or Servings _____

Midafternoon Snack | TIME |

Total Calories or Servings _____

Dinner | TIME |

Total Calories or Servings _____

Nighttime Snack | TIME |

Total Calories or Servings

WORKOUT
Cardio/Walk | TIME | | DURATION |

Strength workout | TIME |

Rate strength of cravings throughout day
(1 being very strong and 10 being no cravings at all):

1   2   3   4   5   6   7   8   9   10

Rate overall mood *(1 being poorest and 10 being best):*

1   2   3   4   5   6   7   8   9   10

Additional comments/notes/questions:

Cycle Watch

Day of cycle *(Comments):*

Season *(Comments):*

Week __ Reshape Day 6

Rate quality of sleep: (*1 being poorest and 10 being best*)

1   2   3   4   5   6   7   8   9   10

Breakfast | TIME |

_____

Total Calories or Servings _____

Midmorning Snack | TIME |

_____

Total Calories or Servings _____

Lunch | TIME |

_____

Total Calories or Servings _____

Midafternoon Snack | TIME |

_____

Total Calories or Servings _____

Dinner | TIME |

_____

Total Calories or Servings _____

Nighttime Snack |TIME| _____ _____

_____

_____

Total Calories or Servings _____

WORKOUT

Cardio/Walk |TIME| _____ |DURATION| _____ _____

....

Strength workout |TIME| _____ _____

_____

Rate strength of cravings throughout day
(1 being very strong and 10 being no cravings at all):

1   2   3   4   5   6   7   8   9   10

Rate overall mood *(1 being poorest and 10 being best):*

1   2   3   4   5   6   7   8   9   10

Additional comments/notes/questions: _____

_____

_____

Cycle Watch

Day of cycle *(Comments):* _____

_____

Season *(Comments):* _____

_____

Week ___ Reshape   Day 7

Rate quality of sleep: *(1 being poorest and 10 being best)*

1   2   3   4   5   6   7   8   9   10

Breakfast   TIME _____

_____

_____

_____

Total Calories or Servings _____

Midmorning Snack   TIME _____

_____

Total Calories or Servings _____

Lunch   TIME _____

_____

_____

_____

Total Calories or Servings _____

Midafternoon Snack   TIME _____

_____

Total Calories or Servings _____

Dinner   TIME _____

_____

_____

_____

_____

Total Calories or Servings _____

Nighttime Snack | TIME | _____

_____

Total Calories or Servings _____

WORKOUT

Cardio/Walk | TIME | | DURATION | _____

_____

Strength workout | TIME | _____

_____

Rate strength of cravings throughout day
(1 being very strong and 10 being no cravings at all):

1   2   3   4   5   6   7   8   9   10

Rate overall mood _(1 being poorest and 10 being best):_

1   2   3   4   5   6   7   8   9   10

Additional comments/notes/questions: _____

_____

Cycle Watch

Day of cycle _(Comments):_ _____

_____

Season _(Comments):_ _____

_____

Week __ Check-In

WEIGHT	
CHEST	
WAIST	
HIPS (AT FULLEST PART)	
LEFT THIGH	
RIGHT THIGH	
LEFT BICEPS	
RIGHT BICEPS	

Overall Weekly Energy Level

(1 = I wish I was still in bed, 10 = I'm like a kid in a candy store)

1   2   3   4   5   6   7   8   9   10

Your Week in Review

Use this space to record any additional thoughts or feelings or to look back on the last couple of days and mark your success on the Belly Melt Diet.

_____

_____

_____

_____

_____

_____

_____

_____

_____

_____

_____

Index

Underscored page references indicate boxed text and sidebars. **Boldface** references indicate photographs.

Crepes
    Toasted Coconut and Banana Crepes, 238
Cross-over bridge, 306, **306**

D

Darkness, for improving sleep, 44–46
Davis, Mary, 42–43, **42**, **43**, 44, 113, 259, **259**
Dawn simulator, 57–58, 66
Decongestants, best time to take, 46
Delayed sleep phase disorder (DSPD), 65–67
Depression, 64, 65, 73, 74, 75, 105, 108, 109, 264,
        328, 329, 333. *See also* Seasonal affective
        disorder (SAD)
Diabetes, 7, 8, 25, 251, 261
    from sleep deprivation, 9, 22, 27, 96, 333
Diets, problems with, 11, 13, 83–84, 89
Dinner
    alcohol with, 94
    guidelines for eating, 325
    recipes for, 188–227
Dips
    Cheesy Lemon-Pepper Dip, 235
    Fresh Fruit with Lime Yogurt Dip, 228
Diurnal rhythms, 5
Doorway inside stretch, 281, **281**
Doorway outside stretch, 282, **282**
Double-knee trunk curl, 296, **296**
Downward dog (yoga pose), 308, **308**
DSPD, 65–67
Dumbbell bench press, 276, **276**
Dumbbell bent row, 277, **277**
Dumbbell heel raise, 289, **289**
Dumbbell lying triceps extension, 280, **280**
Dumbbell side lunge, 288, **288**
Dumbbell squat, 287, **287**
Dumbbell standing cul, 279, **279**
Dumbbell standing press, 278, **278**

E

Edamame
    Edamame Salad with Carrot Ginger Dressing,
        166
Eggplant
    Eggplant Parmesan, 224
Eggs
    Garlic 'n' Herb Vegetable Egg Scramble, 149
    Huevos Rancheros, 158
    Poached Eggs with Parmesan Cheese and
        Spinach, 156
    Spicy Tex-Mex Quiche, 161
    Sweet Potato Hash Brown Eggs, 162
Electronic devices, disrupting sleep, 44, 45, 45,
        325

Endometrial cancer, 77, 261
Energy
    improved, in Belly Melt test panelists, 79, 91,
        125, 337
    from sleep, 20, 27
    walking for, 254
English muffins
    Double-Crunch Peanut Butter and Jelly
        Muffin, 153
    French Onion Tuna Muffin, 164
Estrogen
    bone health from, 262–63
    effect on exercise pain, 257
    effect on sleep, 12, 71, 72, 74
    leptin and, 86
Exercise(s), 249. *See also* Belly Melt Diet
        Workouts; Cardio exercise; Strength
        training; Stretches; Walking; *specific
        exercises*
    of Belly Melt panelists, 43, 79, 90, 113, 125,
        145, 146, 267
    best times for, 250–53, 321, 324
    Kegel, 258
    late-night, myth about, 28
    light therapy promoting, 331
    during menstrual cycle, 257
    motivation for, 256, 258–65
    for reducing cravings, 120
    schedule for, 254
    seasonal effects on, 254–56, 256
    syncing, with circadian rhythms, 249,
        253–54

F

Falafel
    Baked Falafel Sandwiches, 187
    Shepherd's Salad, 167
Fasting, for avoiding jet lag, 335
Fat burning, 256, 321
Fat cells, 24–26
Fatigue, effect on weight, 10, 13
Fat loss, sleep deprivation preventing,
        24
Fats, dietary
    best time to eat, 94–95, 325
    lunchtime craving for, 93
    omega-3 fatty acids, 104
    as sleep disrupter, 54–55
    weight gain from, 88
FEO. *See* Food-entrained oscillator
Figs
    Fig Almond Biscotti, 240
Figure-4 stretch, 290, **290**

Jet lag, 53, <u>69</u>, 87, <u>335</u>

Journal(ing). *See also* Belly Melt Diet Journal
    about PMS-related insomnia, 72
    exercise, 258
    sleep, 67, 68
    time diary, 27, 29

K

Kale
    Pan-Seared Salmon over Kale, 217
Kegel exercises, <u>258</u>
Kiwifruit
    Fresh Fruit with Lime Yogurt Dip, 228

L

Lamb chops
    Grilled Lamb Chops with Tomatoes and Orzo,
      196
Larks
    quiz on, <u>16–17</u>
    temperature fluctuations in, <u>15</u>
Lavender, for inducing sleep, <u>60</u>
Legs-up-the-wall inversion (yoga pose), <u>30</u>, 314,
    314
Legs-up trunk curl, 297, **297**
Lemons
    Greek Lemon and Chicken Soup, 211
    Lemon Almond Cheesecake Parfait, 237
Lentils
    Bulgur Lentil Pilaf with Apple, 226
    Red Lentil Soup, 175
LEO, 5–6
Leptin
    alcohol decreasing, 54
    discovery of, 25
    food clock affecting, 92, 94, 95, 322, 324, 325
    functions of, 11
    hunger cues from, 85–86, <u>86</u>, 100
    injections, ineffectiveness of, <u>98</u>
    premenstrual levels of, 108
    sleep deprivation decreasing, 21–22, 23, 24,
      30, 84, <u>96</u>, <u>97</u>, 334
Letter T stretch, 292, **292**
Lettuce
    Pork Lettuce Wraps, 197
Light cues, 4, 6–7
Light-entrained oscillator (LEO), 5–6
Light exposure
    for jet lag, <u>69</u>
    melatonin production and, 11–12, 40–41, 44,
      45, <u>45</u>, 66
    reducing, for better sleep, 44–46, 325
    for resetting sleep/wake cycle, 321

    for shift workers, 335
    for waking up, 57–58
    weight gain and, 41, 44
Light therapy, <u>64–65</u>, 65, 70, 72, 329–31
Limes
    Chicken Vegetable Soup with Ginger and
      Lime, 176
    Fresh Fruit with Lime Yogurt Dip, 228
Longevity, exercise for, 260–62
Lugo, Idalissa, <u>144–45</u>, **144**, **145**
Lunch
    food choices for, 93, 323
    recipes for, 165–87
    timing of, 94, 323–24

M

Magnesium, 105–6, 107, 109
Mammogram, best time for, <u>71</u>
Mattress, replacing, 49
MBSR, <u>58</u>
Meal plans
    Reset 3-Day, 120, <u>121–23</u>
    Reshape 2-Week, 129, <u>130–43</u>
Meal skipping, increasing ghrelin, 85–86, 87–88,
    89, 92
Meal timing
    in Belly Melt Diet, 96
    effect on hunger hormones, 86–89, 92–95, <u>93</u>,
      128
Measurements, recording, 339, <u>341</u>
Meditation, <u>58</u>
Melatonin
    with advanced sleep phase disorder, 68
    age decreasing, 74
    dawn simulator reducing, 58
    female hormones and, 71
    food sources of, 56, <u>57</u>
    functions of, 11–12
    light exposure and, 11–12, 40–41, 44, 45, <u>45</u>,
      66
    production of, 40, 93, 95, 104, 105, 108, 323,
      325
    tryptophan and, <u>96</u>
Melatonin supplements
    for jet lag, <u>69</u>
    as sleep aid, 53, 65, 67, 68, 70, 72, 338
Menopause, 64, 72–77, <u>86</u>
Menstrual cycle, 64, 106–7
Menstruation, 12, 13, <u>257</u>. *See also* PMDD; PMS
Metabolic syndrome, 8, <u>96</u>
Milk, as sleep aid, 55–56
Miller, Andrea, <u>124–25</u>, **124**, **125**
Mindfulness-based stress reduction (MBSR), <u>58</u>

RLS, 39
Row, row, row your back, 305, **305**
Rowing abs, 304, **304**

S